Last Best Gifts

Last Best Gifts

*Altruism and the Market for
Human Blood and Organs*

KIERAN HEALY

The University of Chicago Press   *Chicago and London*

KIERAN HEALY is assistant professor of sociology at the University of Arizona.

The University of Chicago Press, Chicago 60637
The University of Chicago Press, Ltd., London
© 2006 by The University of Chicago
All rights reserved. Published 2006
Printed in the United States of America

15 14 13 12 11 10 09 08   2 3 4 5

ISBN: 0-226-32235-1 (cloth)
ISBN: 0-226-32237-8 (paper)

Library of Congress Cataloging-in-Publication Data

Healy, Kieran Joseph, 1973–
Last best gifts : altruism and the market for human blood and organs / Kieran Healy.
    p. cm.
  ISBN 0-226-32235-1 (cloth : alk. paper)—ISBN 0-226-32237-8 (pbk. : alk. paper)
   1. Procurement of organs, tissues, etc. 2. Procurement of organs, tissues, etc.—Economic
aspects—United States. 3. Transplantation of organs, tissues, etc.—Economic aspects—United
States. 4. Tissue banks—United States. I. Title.

RD129.5.H43 2006
362.17'84—dc22   2005030538

♾ The paper used in this publication meets the minimum requirements
of the American National Standard for Information Sciences—
Permanence of Paper for Printed Library Materials, ANSI Z39.48-1992.

For my parents,

DERRY AND MARY HEALY

Contents

can have large effects on procurement. These findings are in sharp contrast to the emphasis on individual motives for giving found in both public accounts of donation and much of the research on donation.

Illustrations

Acknowledgments

This book has its deepest roots in a conversation in Cork with Paddy O'Carroll about Richard Titmuss's book *The Gift Relationship,* when I was an undergraduate. It was a typical encounter for both of us: he couldn't remember the book's title (or its author), and I wasn't sharp enough to grasp the substantive point he was making. Later, as a graduate student at Princeton, I was nudged back in the direction of Titmuss by Michèle Lamont. As the project took shape, Paul Starr provided encouragement and advice. Once I began to research and write about exchange in blood and organs, I was lucky to have a superb group of faculty to guide me. Paul DiMaggio's sociological insight and critical acumen is equaled only by his generosity and enthusiasm. The latter never flagged, even when I persistently refused to adopt any of the wholly inappropriate titles he suggested for this book. I benefited many times, too, from Viviana Zelizer's efforts to make me think more deeply and express myself more clearly (and perhaps also more quickly) about this topic. Bruce Western's advice improved this project from its earliest days and his remarkable example as a scholar gave me a target to aim at. Incisive comments from Bob Wuthnow helped give direction to the project at the beginning and shoved it along at a critical stage. And although he had no formal role in supervising my work, Frank Dobbin had a deeper influence on how I went about doing it than he may realize.

Many people have been subjected to different versions of this book in writing or in conversation. Their ideas and criticism have improved it no end, and I am only sorry I cannot hold them responsible for any remaining shortcomings. At Princeton, Courtney Bender, Bethany Bryson, Julian Dierkes, John Evans, Marion Fourcade-Gourinchas, Eszter Hargittai, Jason Kaufman, Erin Kelly, Becky Pettit, Brian Steensland, Steven Tepper, Craig Upright, and Dirk Zorn all helped in many different ways. Thank you. I doubted that I would find another academic community as generous and engaging as I found at Princeton, but happily the University of Arizona's sociology department proved me wrong. In particular, I thank Ron Breiger, Joe Galaskiewicz, Miller McPherson, and Sarah Soule for their guidance and comments. Mark Chaves and Linda Molm each chaired the sociology department while I was writing the book and provided both scholarly advice and practical support. Sherry Enderle and her staff made life easier to manage. A draft of the manuscript was completed while on leave from Arizona at the Social and Political Theory Program in the Australian National University's Research School of Social Sciences. The interdisciplinary environment there helped broaden the scope of the book. Research for this book has been supported at various times by Princeton University, the Woodrow Wilson School of Public and International Affairs, the Noah Cotsen Junior Teaching Fellowship, the National Science Foundation, and the University of Arizona.

Dave Wendler and Neil Dickert kindly shared some of the data analyzed in chapter 3. I am grateful to Ettore Dal Farra for providing detailed information on Italy and for raising some acute questions about the comparative sociology of blood donation in Europe. At various stages I received excellent comments on drafts of chapters from Ed Amenta, Helmut Anheier, Miguel Centeno, and Lynn Spillman. Courtney Bender, Marion Fourcade-Gourinchas, and Brian Steensland read and commented on the last draft of the manuscript. Two anonymous readers for the University of Chicago Press provided very constructive reviews. Thanks also to Doug Mitchell and Tim McGovern at the Press for their enthusiasm and expertise, and to Joel Score for his keen editorial eye.

The data analyses in this book are new, but in several cases earlier versions have appeared as articles. An earlier version of chapter 2 appeared as "Sacred Markets and Secular Ritual in the Organ Transplant Industry," in *The Sociology of the Economy*, edited by Frank Dobbin, 308–31 (New York: Russell Sage, 2004). An earlier version of chapter 5 appeared as "The Emergence of HIV in the U.S. Blood Supply," in *Theory and Society* 28 (1999): 529–58. Parts of chapters 3 and 4 are based on "Altruism as an Organizational Problem," *American Sociological Review* 69 (2004): 387–404 and "Embedded Altruism," *American Journal of Sociology* 105 (2000): 1633–57.

Finally, I want to thank Laurie Paul, but for so many things that there is no hope of covering them all here. By a stroke of terrific good luck, however, she is my wife and so I can go through the list with her in person. I'm also fortunate in that she is an expert in the analysis of counterfactual conditionals. This means she understands much better than me what it means when I say, "This would never have happened if it weren't for you."

ONE

Exchange in Human Goods

For I can raise no money by vile means:
By heaven, I had rather coin my heart,
And drop my blood for drachmas . . .
JULIUS CAESAR 4.3.80–82

There is no production market for human blood and organs. In most parts of the world, it is illegal to sell your
blood and you cannot offer one of your kidneys (or those of
a dead relative) for sale. With the major exception of plasma
in the United States, these goods—all of which are in great
demand—are supplied for free by voluntary donors.

The gift exchange of these goods is unusual enough to
have provoked a long-running though sporadic debate
about its importance. Thanks in part to new possibilities for
commercial trade in human goods opened up by medical
science, and to the growth in for-profit traffic in human
organs and tissue around the world, these arguments have
recently been taken up with renewed vigor in a number of
disciplines.[1] At their core are questions about how and why
the introduction of money affects formerly noncommercial
goods and the social relations that surround them. Is there
something special about the things we reserve for non-
monetary exchange? Does gift exchange have beneficial
effects that market exchange does not?

Although gift giving is the mechanism through which
most blood and organs are collected, it does not happen
everywhere in the same way or to the same extent. The
number of organs and the volume of blood given each year,
both cross-nationally and within particular countries, vary

widely. This fact has not received enough attention in debates about the morality of gift and market exchange in human goods. Yet its implications are striking. If donation simply involves individuals coming forward to give, in much the same way everywhere, why is it so much more common in some countries and regions than in others? Why, for instance, have more than 40 percent of French people given blood but only 16 percent of Norwegians? Why is it that, in the United States, the Midwest yields twice as many organ donors, proportionate to its population, as the South? Does this variation have something to do with the ways the procurement of blood and organs is organized in different places? This is the question I ask in this book.

Put in its broadest terms, my argument is this: to understand this world of goods we must get away from the character and motives of individual donors and look instead to the cultural contexts and organizational mechanisms that provide people with reasons and opportunities to give. Further, we will not understand the social organization of procurement—whether gift based or for profit—if we think there is a simple division between giving and selling. In this introductory chapter, I sketch the theoretical questions at stake and give some background on the specific cases of blood and organs. I then go through some current arguments about commodification and altruism in more detail, with an eye to their relevance to the main question. Finally, I lay out the argument of the book.

Commodifying the Body

Exchange in human goods has grown rapidly over the past thirty years. By human goods I mean body parts or products, from corneas to cadavers; by exchange, any transfer of them, from altruistic donation to for-profit sales. A sense of the size and variety of the "body bazaar" can be found in a recent survey that documents the growth in markets for products as diverse as human hair, leukemia cells, eggs, entire bodies, genetic material, placentas, and brains.[2] As the range and volume of this kind of exchange has grown, so has debate about the form it should take, the risk of exploitation to those involved, and, above all, the proper role of the market. As a rule, the debate is cast as one in which existing relations of selfless, altruistic exchange are threatened with replacement by market-based, for-profit alternatives.

Blood and organ donors give of themselves both figuratively and literally. This mingling of metaphor and reality means that exchange in human goods always has the potential to be more than a simple transfer of products. The U.S. blood supply grew out of the war effort in the 1940s, when the idea of the "nation's blood" was not merely an abstract idea.[3] Blood donations always jump suddenly after disasters as people express their sorrow in a direct and practical way, even though their gift may not always be needed. The long queues outside hospitals and blood centers around the country following the September 11 attacks are the most striking recent example of the moral economy of donation.[4]

While the free gift of blood is seen as an expression of social solidarity, profit-making blood centers have been held up as examples of the depths to which the market can drag a society. In the early 1970s, when the for-profit sale of blood was at its peak in the United States, news features about the squalid world of "ooze for booze" blood centers were common.[5] The international market in blood has proved a powerful symbol of global inequality, too. Douglas Starr describes the fate of the Compañía Centroamericana de Plasmaféresis, a large plasma center in Managua during the Somoza dictatorship that bought its product from poor locals and sold it to companies in the United States. The Somoza family appeared to be involved in the business. After a journalist investigating the plant was killed in suspicious circumstances, the building—known locally as *casa de vampiros*—was attacked by protesters and burned to the ground.[6] Commercial trade in both blood and organs has been seen as the leading edge of a market invasion. Organ procurement has uncomfortable echoes of nineteenth-century body snatching and grave robbing.[7] Policy critics like Jeremy Rifkin and Andrew Kimbrell have argued that technological change in science and medicine, combined with the profit motive, has led companies to turn the human body into a "human body shop."[8] Anthropologists have documented the recent growth of black and gray markets in human organs, in which poor Brazilians, Moldovans, or Filipinos sell their kidneys to wealthy citizens of more developed countries in transactions facilitated by organ brokers.[9] For all these reasons, the sale of human body parts is a standard trope in broader debates about commodification.

The blood supply is generally sufficient for medical needs but is prone to shortages. The demand for organs, by contrast, far outruns the supply. For some commentators, the natural solution to shortages is to introduce a financial incentive—a market price for organs —thus turning donors into paid suppliers. Long considered beyond the pale, the for-profit exchange of blood and organs is now a serious alternative to current policy. For many, however, the prospect of commercial traffic in organs remains disturbing, even obscene, and an altruistic system seems the only morally viable solution. Their intuition is that if the market is going to do damage anywhere, it will be in the exchange of human body products or parts. This area, they believe, is naturally governed by norms of gift giving, altruism, affection, or love, all of which are prime candidates for dissolution or debasement by market institutions.

Commodities are goods produced in order to be traded on markets for profit, and to commodify something is simply to create a market for its exchange where none existed before. But ever since Marx's critique of commodification, the term has connoted much more than this. Marx sees two main things wrong with commodity exchange under capitalism. First, it is exploitative. Marx argues that capitalism cannot exist without a pool of workers who have nothing but their labor power to sell and that the cycle of competition between capitalists will tend to keep wages low.[10] Workers are therefore systematically vulnerable to capitalists in the labor market. Second, this exploitation is obscured because capitalist markets lead people to believe that commodities possess value in their own right, rather than because of the social labor that goes into producing them. This is commodity fetishism.[11] Capitalism is not the only exploitative economic system, but in most others the ultimate source of value—the labor of peasants in a manorial economy, for instance—is at least clear to everyone. Under capitalism, these social relations of production are obscured because people are linked only through the exchange of goods in the market. As a result, the goods appear to have value through some mysterious power of their own.[12]

In one sense, Marx's arguments imply that markets in human goods are no different from other markets. Here, as elsewhere under capitalism, we can expect the vulnerable to be preyed upon. It is not such a big step from exploiting the labor power embodied in workers to exploiting those bodies themselves. Marx's rhetoric, however, shows us that there might be more at stake. His critique of capitalistic commodification is filled with metaphors of bodily violation. The commodity form is "always ready to exchange not only soul, but body, with each and every other commodity."[13] The factory night shift "only slightly quenches the vampire thirst for the living blood of labour,"[14] while apologists for industry insist that "British industry, . . . vampire like, could but live by sucking blood, and children's blood, too."[15] Whereas labor power has "no other repository than human flesh and blood,"[16] the magic of credit means "man himself has been changed into money or money has become incarnate in him. Human individuality, human morality has itself become both an article of commerce and the material in which money exists. Credit no longer analyses money value into money but into human flesh and the human heart."[17] Conversely, the "capitalized blood of children" or other workers moves easily from one country to the next. In all, "capital comes dripping from head to toe, from every pore, with blood and dirt."[18] In considering trade in human blood and organs, then, we find ourselves facing a *literal* market in the very things Marx used as metaphors of capitalistic excess. Horror at the prospect of wholly commodified bodies is built into the foundational critique of capitalist society. We should not be surprised, then, when people see these markets as a confirmation of Marx's intuitions about the insatiability of capitalism.

Marx presented a comprehensive critique of capitalism as a whole, and this is not the place to assess its merits or detail its difficulties. But the problems he identified—systematic exploitation and the atomizing, socially destructive nature of market exchange—are, though often in more refined or narrowly targeted forms, still central to contemporary debates.[19] Critics worry that, by allowing market logic to dictate the terms of an exchange, we risk losing something important. Markets reduce different ways of valuing things to one dimension, measured in money. They encourage us to treat people as means rather than ends. They erode our desire to carry out principled actions unmotivated by profit. They undermine altruistic action—whether heroic or mundane—by rendering it unintelligible. (Why do something for free when you could be paid for it?) They break up social relations, networks, or forms of organization and replace them with ersatz equivalents devoid of depth and meaning.[20] It is also often argued that commodification can have negative effects both on the goods being traded and the people who exchange them.[21] Goods can be debased by money, as, for instance, when someone tries to buy an award or an academic degree. In the same way, people can be corrupted by money, as they come to act only out of self-interest or for profit, and treat others as means to their own ends.

Recent commentators are much less likely than Marx to believe that all goods and actions are equally susceptible to the market's dangers. It is hard to see how commodifying the exchange of, say, paper clips would do anything to debase the paper clips themselves. And it is easy to think of cases where self-interest is an uncontroversially appropriate motive, as when one fends off an attacker. Indeed, as Jon Elster points out, while we can imagine a (nasty) world where everyone is always and only self-interested, a world populated only by pure altruists is harder to conceive. It might be possible for some people to always and only care for the welfare of others, but this could not be true of everyone. Accepting assistance means putting yourself first at least some of the time, and in this sense altruism is parasitic on self-interest.[22] As for the moral dangers posed by commodification (as opposed to mere self-interest), few if any argue that trying to make an honest living in business is an inherently debasing activity that entails being corrupted by money. There is a distinction between profit making and profiteering.

This raises the question of where to draw the line. Goods will not conveniently classify themselves for us: There is little point in "searching fruitlessly for the magic distinction between commodities and other sorts of things."[23] (To think this distinction is built into goods is just another kind of commodity fetishism.) We can roughly distinguish three orientations to commodification. Some things are uncontroversially commodities and we do not worry about their marketability at all. In other cases, commodification is acknowledged as a problem—something that in principle ought not to happen—but corrective responses are possible; a certain amount of it may even be seen as inevitable and tolerable. In the final case, the problem is much more severe: commodification is thought to undermine basic distinctions or sacred values or to threaten social institutions that have powerful defenders.

What kinds of things provoke this last response? It turns out that many intuitively compelling examples of commodification involve, not tangible goods or products in the usual sense, but a social relationship. Depending on the particular relationship, this sort of commodification may be thought to be especially pernicious. Friendship, for instance, is a social tie that is not supposed to be instrumental. Trying to purchase a friend, the argument goes, shows that the buyer (or seller) just doesn't understand what friendship is. Whatever you are getting for your money, ipso facto it cannot be friendship. Goods like friendship, love, and respect by definition cannot be brought to market. When we see items or services for sale bearing those labels, we are really looking at some ersatz or debased alternative, not the good itself.

Michael Walzer's influential catalog of "blocked exchanges" is a list of goods he claims are in this sense naturally and properly outside the sphere of monetary exchange.[24] It does not include many items that you could put in a shop window, apart from human beings. Instead, it is made up mainly of social relations and institutions: he procscribes the sale of political influence, freedom of speech, marriage, criminal justice, and so on. The commodification of political influence, merit, justice, and the like prompts charges of corruption. Indeed, sales of these goods have well-established names: graft, nepotism, simony, bribery. In many of these cases (the pursuit of political office, for instance) we wearily expect money to be present, even if we might prefer to keep it out.

Other goods seem to have a different character. The threat of commodification provokes especially strong reactions where aspects of persons (and their social relationships) that are supposed to be intimate or sacred are made to yield marketable goods or services. Within the household, for instance, money mixes with domestic relations in complicated ways. People frequently end up in court as a result. Social scientists and legal scholars have recently begun to pay serious attention to how money works in these intimate relations.[25] Women's domestic and reproductive labor is typically embedded in the institution of the family, but it also has the potential to be a marketable service. The most common good that is both intimate (usually embedded in affect-laden social relations) and marketable (capable of being separated from a particular individual and sold commercially) is domestic labor. In the 1960s and '70s, proposals to commodify housework often provoked strong reactions, as today do arguments about the growth of markets in child care.[26]

Blood and organs can be thought of as tangible counterparts to these intimate yet marketable social relationships. They are literally part of oneself but can now be turned into discrete, marketable items. The same anxiety-provoking questions—about the place of money in theory and in practice, its role in exchange, and its potential to corrupt people or debase social relationships—are raised in both cases. But unlike a social relationship, you really could put a kidney in a shop window, which makes the prospect of debased exchange seem that much more real.

Do we see these negative outcomes in practice? Equally important, is the implied alternative—exchange governed by norms of gift giving or altruism—as straightforward as it seems? Empirical research is thin. There are few sociological studies of the blood supply and even fewer of the organ industry. At the same time, the blood and organ procurement industry has changed enormously over the last thirty years. Even though the supply still depends on free gifts, tissue procurement and distribution systems are by now remarkably complex. As a rule, they are not yet commercialized at the point of procurement, but the supply is managed in ways that make commonsense understandings of donation seem naïve. We need a way to think about the relationship between those who give (or sell) human goods and those who receive (or buy) them.

Four Arguments about Incentives and Actions

Arguments about the process of commodification and the effects of market exchange are closely related to our ideas about people's motives for their actions. Promarket rhetoric emphasizes the ability of markets to maximize individual utility and collective welfare in a decentralized fashion. Antimarket rhetoric focuses on what for-profit exchange will do to us as human beings: markets will corrupt our motives, diminish our moral worth, appeal to our basest desires, lead us to see others as means rather than ends, and so on. Every account of the market and its effects rests on some sort of theory of what people's motives and desires are or ought to be, and of what money will do to them. There are many such theories, and they go in and out of fashion. This is not the place to present or evaluate all of them. Instead, I will focus on recent research that has tried to pin down this relationship more precisely. The approaches I discuss differ in method, but each tries to get at the role of money and monetary incentives in people's decision making.

Recent discussions of commodification, altruism, and the market draw on one of four contrasting views about the relationship between people's motives and their actions: (1) People are rationally motivated by incentive systems. (2) People adapt their motives to the incentive system. (3) Incentive systems can be subordinated to people's motives. (4) People are culturally constrained to give certain accounts of their actions.

People Are Rationally Motivated by Incentives

This is the easiest approach to describe. It is also the most clearly worked out, most frequently criticized, and most rhetorically successful. Expected-utility theory says that people are motivated by self-interest and have a complete, transitive, continuous set of preferences that allow them to choose between different bundles of goods and services. In general, markets enable goods to flow to those who value them most highly, as measured by their willingness to pay. Free markets are the most efficient way to allocate goods because the equilibrium of supply and demand maximizes welfare, defined as the sum of consumer and producer surplus.

The theory of rationality that underlies these ideas is quite thin.[27] It makes relatively few assumptions about what people are like, but the assumptions that are made have far-reaching implications. Of the arguments presented here it is the only one that does not see money or the market as themselves having any particular effects on people. Money is a neutral medium. In theory it is a way of expressing value in an easily calculable way. In practice it facilitates the exchange of goods. Money does not corrupt or ennoble those who use it; the market is just a way of bringing buyers and sellers together. It promotes the general welfare through an unexpectedly elegant process of decentralized allocation by the invisible hand.[28]

The ostensible neutrality of money and the automatic action of the market may be carried over to the self-presentation of those who subscribe to the theory. Economists sometimes think of themselves as presenting technical results beyond the reach of normative debates, thanks both to the features of their theory and to its apparently positive concept of rationality. This belief is not really true, but it has two important implications. First, rational self-interest is allowed to serve as the default model of action in many policy debates. Second, the presumed technical neutrality of economics can be parlayed into moral authority and thus becomes a rhetorical asset.[29]

From this perspective, a market for blood or organs should be much like any other market. There may be some altruists who would not give their organs away if a market for them existed. But our experience with other goods strongly suggests that creating a market for, say, kidneys would—if the incentives were right—result in a larger supply, even if most of the altruistic suppliers dropped out. Such markets are illegal at present, but those who advocate them argue that this will surely change sooner or later. As blood and especially organ shortages become more acute, the pressure of demand will lead the market to emerge as the obvious solution. The simplest blood and organ markets would involve direct contracts between willing buyers and sellers, with perhaps some state regulation to ensure the quality of the products. But this is only one of several possibilities. A market in organs need not involve people hawking their kidneys in classified ads or on eBay. Some kind of indirect reimbursement—a health insurance premium reduction, for example, or a futures market of some sort—might do just as well, while bypassing the concerns of the squeamish.[30]

People Adapt Their Motives to the Incentives

If we suspect that people are not simply rational utility maximizers, the relationship between monetary incentives and individual motives becomes more complicated and our theory less elegant. For instance, it may be that not everybody is selfish, or at least not all the time. If there are altruists in a population, then the presence of money rewards will discourage rather than encourage them to act. Richard Titmuss made this case for blood. He suggested that if a blood supply runs on cash incentives, then altruistic suppliers will be driven out and be replaced by selfish ones.[31] But because he wrote as though people were either egoists or altruists, Titmuss really just replicated the economistic view of action with a morally disapproving spin. The egoists beat the altruists, and this is bad for everyone. (In chapter 5 we will see that things are more complicated than Titmuss thought.)

Bruno Frey's formulation of this idea is more interesting.[32] He conducted a survey of Swiss citizens who were to decide whether they wanted a nuclear waste dump in their area. (The waste dump proposal was a real proposition, not a hypothetical experiment.) Slightly more than 50 percent of the respondents were prepared to have the waste dump in their backyards, so to speak, even though a large majority (80 percent) knew what the risks were. Respondents were then told that the Swiss government was offering substantial monetary compensation to the residents of the host communities.[33] The rate of consent dropped by half. Frey suggests that the offer of money "crowded out" other motives, such as civic virtue, that had motivated a majority to agree to the proposal without any tangible incentive. Unlike Titmuss, Frey does not distinguish between born egoists and born altruists. Rather, he suggests that people will respond in kind to the incentives they are offered. The point is not simply that bad incentives lead to perverse or unhappy outcomes as individuals make rational choices in the light of those incentives. Rather, actors may assess themselves and their choices using the model of action implied by the system. In Frey's terms, an incentive system designed for knaves will cause people to behave like knaves. Each system will get the people it deserves.

There are several versions of this view. They can be distinguished from one another by the degree to which the authors think that people's motives will be debased by the introduction of monetary incentives. Michael Walzer's early, influential formulation argued that different goods exist in different spheres and that we try to keep the metrics associated with these spheres from leaking into one another.[34] The trend in the more recent literature has been away from this idea. But many commentators are unwilling to give up the idea that money tends to have a corrupting influence on people and their relationships. Margaret Radin's work on commodification is a good example. She rejects Walzer's argument and acknowledges that many relationships are "incompletely commodified" without a great deal of harm being done to them. Many relations or exchanges have a market-oriented aspect, but they will generally have many nonmarket features as well. This leads to the optimistic idea that "the values of personhood and community pervasively interact with the market and alter many things from their pure free-market form."[35]

Still, Radin worries about the power of the market. In particular, she argues that if we insist on talking about all aspects of our society using the rhetoric of the market, we will end up being unable to think about it in other terms: "I don't mean to deny that the rhetoric of economics is frequently useful as one among the many ways we can think about relationships and behavior. I am arguing that something important to humanity is lost if market rhetoric becomes (or is considered to be) the sole rhetoric of human affairs, excluding other kinds of understanding." She suggests that we need various kinds of legal regulation in order to stop this from happening.[36] Radin transposes Frey's argument from internal motivations to cultural discourse and suggests that, in the absence of legal constraints, market talk will crowd out other ways of understanding ourselves. Her concerns are supported by empirical evidence that learning about theories of rational utility maximization, by taking Econ 101, for instance, tends to make people more selfish.[37]

When applied to the case of human goods, this view suggests that we get what we wish for. If we talk of blood as if it were a commodity, then people will come to commodify it in practice. By instituting a market for blood or organs, people orient themselves toward these goods in a new way. The rational calculus of costs and benefits comes to override alternative ways of thinking about the value of what is being exchanged.

Incentive Systems Can Be Subordinated to People's Motives

Frey is concerned that the introduction of money crowds out people's better motives. Viviana Zelizer rejects the general idea that money has the inherent power to do this. Rather than being slaves to money, she argues, people are a good deal smarter than it. People use different payment systems and exchange tokens to express and define different social relations.[38] Zelizer focuses mainly on the ways that people evade the supposedly homogenizing effects of money by earmarking it in different ways. Her historical research shows that even as the American state became increasingly successful at eliminating the variety of unofficial coinage and currency that had circulated in the nineteenth century, people came up with new ways to distinguish kinds of money for their own purposes. Thus, "the forms of monetary earmarking multiplied just as official money became *more* uniform and generalized."[39]

Zelizer and Frey are not talking about quite the same thing. Zelizer wants to show that money is not a neutral, homogeneous medium of exchange. She does not directly address the effects of money as an incentive. Rather, she begins with the idea that people are involved in many different social relationships and then goes on to show how they use money to mark and express those relations. But it is not difficult to see how her ideas might be extended and applied to the question of motivation. Insofar as people share conventions for earmarking—that is, as long as they know how to "read" the underlying social relationship expressed by the form of payment—an offer to enter into some *new* relationship, encoded in a particular payment token, will be easy to understand. They will be able to choose different payment conventions to express different sorts of motivations to act. And as Frey's work suggests, how people read these offers will inform how they respond. An offer of cash compensation from the government suggests one kind of relationship between the state and its citizens, one that the Swiss were quite suspicious of. It looked to them like the government was trying to buy them off. But a different form of payment—a commitment to building new schools, say, or some other form of indirect investment—might have been interpreted differently. Frey does not explore this possibility. By extending Zelizer's ideas, we can speculate that although the physical exchange of a good or service can easily take place within many different social relationships, different relationships will tend to commit the parties to different bundles of motives and expectations.

Zelizer herself does not argue explicitly along these lines, but this idea is consistent with her emphasis on the constitutive role of social relationships in distinguishing kinds of payment tokens and social obligations in different circumstances. When it comes to exchange in human goods, Zelizer's approach suggests that people will not be opposed a priori to payments or reimbursement for the time and effort they take, say, to donate blood. But the form the reimbursement takes will be very important, and the wrong choice by the collection agency might provoke a strongly negative reaction. Similarly, it might not be difficult for the families of organ donors to accept a payment in connection with their decision to donate. But because the form of the payment will mark the kind of social relationship established by the transaction, the organ procurer must tread carefully. A further consequence of these ideas is that the shape of a transaction, and how it is explained or accounted for, is vitally important to those involved and may determine whether the transaction happens at all.

People's Accounts of Their Actions Are Culturally Constrained

The fourth view is somewhat similar to Radin's argument about market rhetoric. In a number of books, Robert Wuthnow has explored how Americans think and talk about money, selfishness, and altruism.[40] He finds that it is difficult to make sense of the idea that people have clear motives for acting in specific circumstances. Instead of being motivated by a consistent underlying principle of selfishness or altruism, or by some stable set of preferences, people can cite many different reasons for why they volunteer, give money to charity, or work so hard at their jobs. In fact, there are *too many* good reasons available. Any one of them would be sufficient. This excess of reasons causes people to avoid accounting for their actions in terms of motives in the first place. They prefer to "situationalize" their actions "by telling stories that embed values in specific contexts, that frame principles as particulars. . . . Accounts of our motives, when all is said, are basically stories—highly personalized stories, not assertions of high-flown values but formulaic expressions of ourselves."[41] People prefer description to motive and like to emphasize how they just happened to get involved in something rather than give the impression that they are somehow deserving of praise.

Wuthnow tells a subtle story about the rules that organize how people talk about their own actions. Of particular interest here are the examples he presents of people shying away from altruistic explanations for their actions. Altruism is not culturally plausible. If someone appears to act in an altruistic way, we may suspect that they are really furthering their own ends. It is not just that we are cynical about other people's motives. Perhaps more significantly, we will often account for our own actions in self-interested terms, even when an unselfish explanation would be more truthful. We may even be more willing to engage in unselfish behavior if we can pretend that we are motivated by self-interest.[42]

Paradoxically, organ donation provides a particularly good example of this cultural suspicion of altruism. Occasionally, someone will approach their doctor or an organ procurement organization and express a desire to donate a kidney, while they are alive, to someone in need. Not to anyone in particular (like a sibling or spouse, as happens with most living donors), just to one of the many thousands of people they know desperately need a transplant. Such an action, on the face of it, is pure altruism of a quite remarkable kind. The donor will not meet the recipient of their organ, and there is no external motivation whatsoever to give. But even though the transplant community continuously emphasizes its gratitude to donor families, and often calls them heroes, reaction to these potential donors has been different. Until recently, transplant coordinators would not consider such an operation. Not only have doctors been reluctant to encourage such donations, but their initial reaction has been to suspect that the would-be donors are mentally ill. In newspaper accounts of transplants involving such donors, doctors commonly note that they questioned the donor's motives and were allowed to proceed only after the donor passed a rigorous psychological evaluation.[43]

———

What should we make of these four versions of the link between motives and actions? The first two are oriented toward the individual and are quite strongly cognitive: they make claims about what goes on in people's heads when money incentives are offered to them and lead to normative questions about commodification. For economists, the problem of how to value things is already solved and built into the assumptions of utility theory. The question then is why there *aren't* markets for blood and organs, given their superiority in allocating goods. In philosophy and law, these questions can be answered in three main ways: by relying on a theory that says what we should value and how, by having some way of calculating the good and bad consequences of commodification, or by appealing to societal values to tell us which exchanges should not be subject to the market. Although legal and philosophical work does consider empirical evidence about how people use money and how exchange is organized, its main concern is to develop normative arguments about whether and to what extent we ought to limit people's exposure to the market.

In contrast, sociological work looks more closely at the cultural and institutional basis of what is often called simply "the logic of the market." Zelizer shows that people are creative with money—they aren't simply corrupted by or enslaved to it. Neither is it a merely neutral medium of exchange. Her work broadens the debate because it shows people have more room to act, in particular to use money to draw distinctions between kinds of social relations, than other discussions credit them with. These findings support arguments of the sort made by Elizabeth Anderson and Margaret Radin, in that they show people expressing qualitatively different sorts of value in a wide variety of social relationships. But they undercut those arguments, too, by showing how flexible people can be when it comes to using money in social relationships, even intimate ones like sex or family.

Wuthnow similarly moves us away from questions of individual motive and character. This is true even though his research is filled with the voices of interviewees accounting for their charitable acts and explaining how they think about money. Wuthnow shows that people are reluctant to speak about themselves and money in particular ways. It's not that people don't want to admit that they're motivated by money or success—that's what the American dream is all about, after all. They have no general conviction that markets are a bad thing. Rather, they usually don't want to be pinned down to some specific set of selfish motives. Even when they are acting out of self-interest they generally do not want to appear *calculating,* especially with regard to friends or relatives. But people don't want to seem too saintly either, so they avoid accounting for their actions in altruistic terms, even when such accounts would be plausible. Instead, they tell stories, often built around chains of contingencies, about how they ended up volunteering their time or doing a particular job, or spending so much time at work. When they do appeal to more general standards, they often rely on language produced and refined by organizations specializing in voluntary work. I argue for an approach that focuses first on the institutions that organize exchange, rather than the self-interested or altruistic motives of individuals. This does not mean we do away with individuals and incentives, or with reasons for giving. We have a good social psychology of altruism that explains a great deal about how people choose to give and how they come to think of themselves as the sort of person who volunteers their time, contributes their money, or donates their blood.[44] But a social-psychological view is not enough to account for the variation we see over time, across organizations, and between countries. Individual motives play out within social contexts organized around particular conceptions of the relationship between donors and recipients—the gift relationship.

Gifts and Markets

What is a gift? What does a gift relationship entail? The classic answers to these questions were given by Marcel Mauss and Bronislaw Malinowski.[45] A long tradition of scholarship and empirical study in anthropology pursues these questions in great detail.[46] Here I will focus on the Maussian insight that a gift is something much more general than a present wrapped up and given on a special occasion. Rather, gift exchange can involve "any object or service, utilitarian or superfluous. . . . 'Gift' does not identify either the object or service itself, or the forms and ceremonies of giving and getting. Instead, what makes a gift is the relationship within which the transaction occurs."[47] In gift exchange, transactions are *obligatory,* the goods exchanged are unique or *inalienable,* and the exchange partners are *related* in some way beyond the specific transaction.[48] Contrast this with an archetypal market relationship. In the market, exchanges are voluntary or formally free (no one is forced to buy or sell), the goods exchanged are fungible, and exchange partners are linked only by the contract governing that particular transaction.

Gift exchange is obligatory in two senses. There is a general expectation that everyone (in the relevant group) ought to participate in the transaction, and in particular cases the exchange of gifts recreates the expectation of future participation. This kind of exchange can be thought of in utilitarian terms, with individuals always assessing how much they owe to others and finding ways to place people in their debt. This was Malinowski's view: "sooner or later an equivalent repayment or counter-service" would always be demanded by the giver.[49] Mauss acknowledged this aspect of giving, noting that "the unreciprocated gift . . . makes the person who has accepted it inferior, particularly when it has been accepted with no thought of returning it."[50] But this obligation to reciprocate also expresses the continuing existence of a particular relationship between the parties, and, as James Carrier puts it, this is not just a matter of profit and loss within the exchange:

Doubtless, if one party to a gift relationship feels regularly and unjustly slighted, he or she will consider ending the relationship. But this does not mean that the transactor is calculating debts and credits, emotional or material. . . . Instead, the repeated imbalance itself marks a repeated violation of the obligation to give, receive and repay in that relationship, and hence marks the end of that relationship as it had been.[51]

The other two dimensions of gift exchange reinforce this point. Gifts are not fungible or anonymous items but rather are inalienable, in the sense that they carry the identity of the giver with them. Gifts are "followed around by their former owner, and they follow him also," in Mauss's phrase.[52] This of course is not some magical quality that gifts mysteriously have. Mauss means that gifts are particular objects rather than anonymous items and that their particularity comes from their tie to a specific person.[53] The third dimension of gift exchange highlights these persistent social ties between exchange partners. Giver and receiver are aware of this relationship during and after the transaction. We can see that each aspect of the gift relationship is implicated in the others: obligations presuppose social relationships; exchanges within relationships express the social identities of the partners and re-create the obligations; gifts renew social ties between individuals and further develop their relationship to one another. This is what Mauss means when he says that gift exchange is a "total" social phenomenon, where "all kinds of institutions are given expression at one and the same time."[54]

Putting gift and market exchange side by side is a good way to bring out the distinctive qualities of each. They work on different principles, but we should be clear about what this will mean in practice. Although Mauss himself saw gift and commodity exchange as belonging to different social worlds, it is more useful to think of them as tendencies that can be found together to greater or lesser degrees in the same society. For instance, we should not think that the presence of money automatically means that gift exchange is impossible or has been driven out by the market. (This is one of the main lessons of the recent economic sociology discussed in the previous section.) Circuits of gift giving persist and thrive alongside the market. Moreover, long-term relationships *within* the market may have many of the features of gift exchange, despite the fact that its transactions are nominally governed by contracts.

In important ways, exchange in human goods does not fit well into the classical account of the gift relationship. The key difference is that it cannot be a face-to-face transaction. Blood and organs must be collected and distributed by complex organizations. And yet, in part because of the powerful potential of human goods to express social solidarity, the "gift template" still governs the exchange, and each dimension of the gift relationship is present in the practice of blood and organ donation. The coordinating organizations work to elicit donations from donors, to elaborate the meaning of the donation, and to specify the nature of the gift and the obligations that flow from it. This work involves both logistical and cultural effort. The result is a practical system of procurement and distribution but also a moral order of exchange. How successful these organizations are at managing each aspect of this process—and whether the varying demands they face are reconcilable—is the subject of the rest of the book.

An Overview of the Book

Organizations procuring blood and organs create and sustain their donor pools by providing opportunities to give and by producing and popularizing accounts of what giving means. This means that the structure and practices of these organizations play a larger role in our understanding of blood and organ donation than much of the debate on the relative merits of self-interest and altruism would lead us to believe. Procurement organizations do their work in different ways and with different resources to hand. As a result, some are more successful than others. There is substantial variation in procurement rates for both blood and organs, and while some of this variation comes from the individual qualities of donors or features of the social environment much of it has its source in the structure, scope, and strategies of the organizations in charge of the supply. Organizations do not simply manipulate donors more or less effectively: they are themselves affected by the exchange relations they institutionalize, and this can have important consequences. The conception of the gift relationship promoted by procurement organizations affects how the organizations themselves understand their own interests and, as we shall see, how they respond to crises in the supply.

When I say organizations produce and sustain altruism I mean that they have large effects on the volume of blood and the number of organs procured each year, but also that they shape our *ideas* about altruism and donation by producing accounts of what it means to be a donor. Chapter 2 traces the emergence of the cultural account of organ donation in the United States from the late 1970s to the 1990s. As organ donation became more common, transplant advocates worked to convince the public that it was a morally worthwhile idea. By publicizing a specific set of arguments for donation, lobbying politically, and working to placate or sideline their critics, they helped make donation a socially acceptable choice in the face of sudden bereavement. I show how this process resembles the historical debate over the growth of the life insurance market, another good that was initially controversial. If we follow the course of the public debate about transplants over a twenty-five-year period, we will see that the range of responses to the new technology narrows over time. The standard account of organ donation represents a consensus produced through the professional efforts of transplant advocates.

This consensus was not fixed, however. As the demand for organs continued to grow, serious discussion of financial incentives for organ donors became more and more common. I trace the rise of "market talk" about organ donation and show how it has gradually become more acceptable to talk about organ procurement in this way. But there is a large gap between the straightforwardly profit-oriented proposals to introduce a market for organs and the more sophisticated payment systems thought by many to be practical solutions. Simple "cash for organs" markets of the kind most feared and criticized in standard accounts of commodification are not widely advocated today (though they were the first proposals to be articulated). When it comes to making policy, the most successful market advocates are also the ones most sensitive to sociological questions about the expressiveness of payment tokens and the meaning of the exchange relations they imply, even though they usually do not draw attention to this fact themselves.

Organizations produce cultural accounts of donation, but mostly they do the hard work of procuring blood and organs from donors, often in difficult circumstances. Inevitably they tackle the problem of finding donors in different ways, and this leads to variation in the rates of donation that we observe. Chapters 3 and 4 explore the effects that organizations have, both on the size of the blood and organ supply and on the characteristics of the donors who provide the goods.

Chapter 3 asks why some organ procurement organizations (OPOs) manage to collect more organs than others. Many things affect organ procurement rates, from individual decisions to sign a donor card, to county mortality rates, to state road-safety laws. Sorting them out with the available data is difficult. This chapter quantifies the structural and organizational forces at work in the procurement process. On the structural side, I show how differences between the service populations of OPOs affect their procurement rates. The characteristics of these populations—such as their density, racial composition, and poverty rate—have strong effects. In terms of organization, I measure the role played by the size and operating budget of OPOs, their logistical scope, and their procurement policies and strategies. This analysis takes us away from the image of the individual donor motivated by generosity, an image that these organizations have themselves done much to create and popularize. It does not do away with that image or render it meaningless. But it does show that it would be impossible for individuals to act so generously in the absence of these organizations and that, in spite of the variety of individual motives and choices, structural and institutional patterns explain most of the variation in procurement rates.

An important difference between blood and organ donation is that blood is relatively easy to donate and can be given regularly. Nevertheless, very few eligible donors ever give. Is this because there are not many altruists in the world or because blood collection organizations could be doing a better job? Chapter 4 tackles this issue from a comparative, cross-national perspective. The empirical question is, how does the social organization of the blood supply affect the quantity of blood collected and the character of the donors who give it? As with the organ supply within the United States, I begin with the observation that the amount of blood collected in Europe varies a great deal across different countries. If altruism was a strictly individual characteristic, we should not expect donation rates to differ between countries as much as they do. Drawing on data about the organization of the European Union's blood supply and patterns of donation across Europe, I show that different "collection regimes" not only affect the size and shape of the donor pool (i.e., the volume collected and the sociodemographic makeup of the donor population) but also shape the *character* of donation, determining in part what sort of an activity it is and what it means. For instance, students are less likely than average to have ever given blood, except in countries where the Red Cross is in charge of the supply. In those countries, students are significantly more likely to have given. The explanation is organizational: the Red Cross effectively recruits students, while state-run or independent blood-banking systems do not seems to do so as effectively. Again, the more general argument is that our understanding of altruistic action is greatly improved by taking a comparative, organizational perspective.

Chapters 2 through 4 treat the altruism involved in the procurement and exchange of blood and organs as an outcome. Variation in the size and composition of the donor pool is the result of differences between the organizations that manage the supply of blood or organs. Chapter 5 takes the argument a step further. There I argue that, in some circumstances, the exchange relations that organizations sustain through their public accounts of donation can have important effects on decision making by the organizations themselves. As the moral expectations associated with different kinds of exchange relation become institutionalized, they can affect how organizations respond to new information in their environment. Chapter 5 examines what happened to the U.S. blood supply when a new disease was discovered within it. Why did the organizations in control of different parts of the blood supply react as they did to the emergence of HIV in the early 1980s? They did not all respond in the same way to the crisis, even though they all had the same information about it and, in retrospect, there were some steps all of them should have taken. I argue that the exchange relationships linking blood suppliers and recipients to collection organizations shaped what these organizations did. The obligations attached to these relationships affected the way blood collection organizations understood their interests and, as a consequence, how they reacted to uncertainty about HIV. I also show that the effects of gift-based and profit-based relationships were not what the conventional wisdom predicted.

In the concluding chapter, I draw together these empirical findings and ask what they can tell us about the future of exchange in human goods. As demand for organs increases and new secondary markets for human tissues emerge, the ultimate source of almost all these goods remains freely given gifts. I ask whether changes in the logistics of procurement—increasing efforts to procure donors efficiently, the pathway followed by donated tissues, the multiple uses to which whole blood is immediately put—are undermining the moral order of exchange, encapsulated in the idea of the "gift of life," that procurement organizations have worked so hard to establish. The gift exchange of blood and organs has proved surprisingly robust, but I argue that the short-run logistical demands placed on procurement organizations are in tension with the cultural account of donation that they have produced over the long run. The public conception of exchange in human goods, and especially organ donation, is at odds with rapidly growing and increasingly lucrative secondary markets in human tissues.

———

When arguing about the ethics of blood or organ sales, it is tempting to believe that we know what the outcome would be if a market for kidneys was created. Perhaps it would run smoothly along lines prescribed by a straightforward account of the economics of a commodity market. Or we might be instinctively horrified at the prospect and feel that profitable exchange in kidneys is neither morally nor socially viable. Commodification is often presented as a semiautomatic process of debasement or deterioration. Voluntary giving becomes, by implication, a safer, less exploitative way to exchange goods that should not be priced by the market. Contemporary bioethical debate about blood and organ donation focuses overwhelmingly on the moment of individual choice, the decision to give or sell, and its moral implications are measured in terms of the amount of autonomy possessed by the donor and the degree to which their consent is informed.[55] Sometimes the absence of money is taken as the best indicator of an absence of coercion, even though gift exchanges are often a conduit for power. Studies of how goods are measured, compared, and transferred in practice—the sociology of commensuration—provide a corrective to this tendency by asking where standards for choice and comparison come from. Commensuration is "the expression or measurement of characteristics normally represented by different units according to a common metric."[56] Two things are incommensurable, roughly, when they "cannot be aligned along a single metric without doing violence to our considered judgments about how these goods are best characterized."[57] Of central interest from a sociological point of view are the "social technologies" of measurement and comparison that take unique or heterogenous items and make them comparable according to some metric.[58] In parallel fashion, a clear understanding of the organizational efforts that keep items *out* of the market is central to understanding the structure of exchange in human goods. "Donation" suggests a system where gifts are unconditionally given and gratefully received. But research on markets and actual systems of gift exchange shows a more complex reality than the stylized versions often found in public debates about commodification and altruism.

Organizations produce logistical opportunities to give, thereby finding and recruiting donors. Accounts of this process are put together informally by participants and more systematically by organizations with people to motivate. Donors, doctors, and beneficiaries write books, publish articles, and give talks to help spread their message. Similarly, the organizations have problems that their staffs must deal with, so they invent schemes, lobby lawmakers, and write professional guidelines to help solve them. But because stories propagate as accounts and solutions establish themselves as institutionalized scripts, they may grow beyond their origins and can begin to shape the exchanges they describe. The study of altruism generally, and the case of human goods in particular, has neglected these processes and focused instead on heroic individual altruists.[59] Research framed in this way can offer effective counterexamples to the strongest claims about all-pervasive selfishness, but in the process it accepts too much of the received wisdom about the nature of giving behavior and the dangers money poses to it.

Students of cross-national variation in economic institutions have repeatedly shown that different countries and regions institutionalize their own distinctive varieties of capitalism, and that what people mean by "self-interest, rightly understood" varies with these institutions. The institutional basis of altruism has been less closely examined, and the active production both of opportunities for altruism and the social identities that go along with them is a neglected topic. The voluntary donation of human goods is an organizational accomplishment. Procurement organizations with resource problems to solve must first find donors as effectively as they can, then manage them by elaborating and institutionalizing a conception of gift exchange that makes individual donations meaningful, while making large-scale procurement possible.

TWO

Making a Gift

Over the past thirty years, organ transplantation has been transformed from an experimental therapy of last resort into a common medical procedure. As a consequence, demand for human organs has increased sharply and the number of people waiting for transplants exceeds the number of available organs by a factor of about ten. A network of organ procurement organizations (OPOs) has grown up to collect and distribute organs in the United States. Along with the government and the medical profession, these organizations have worked to increase the supply, both by collecting as many organs as possible and by convincing more people to become organ donors. Convincing the public of the rightness of organ donation has not always been easy. Organ procurement has the potential to be controversial, I argue, because it crosses two sacred social boundaries. It introduces a utilitarian calculation at the time of death, and it threatens to place a cash value on human life.

I argue that transplant advocates developed a specific cultural account of donation to fix these breaches. An account is a coherent body of reasons and evaluations that can be used to explain and legitimate some practice or activity.[1] The cultural account of donation can be seen in the promotional materials and professional handbooks of OPOs, in books and memoirs about organ donation, and in the media coverage of donation issues. It amounts to a repertoire of reasons, motives, and stories—a set of "feeling rules" for the experience of organ donation, in Arlie Hochschild's phrase.[2] The features of a gift relationship can be found in it, elaborated in a fashion appropriate to organ donation. I argue that this account is prescriptive rather than descriptive: it presents the ideal experience, what one ought to feel in these circumstances rather than what many people actually experience. Evidence for this comes from a number of facts about the discourse: advocates of organ donation tried more than one approach before settling on the current rules, themes found in earlier sources are not found in later ones, the popular account focuses on atypical cases, and documentary and interview evidence shows a much wider spectrum of feeling about organ donation than the official account suggests.

This cultural work has tended to be glossed over in standard debates about commodification, but it is central to understanding how this new, potentially threatening practice has come to be accepted and encouraged. Arguments over commodification try to decide what is and what is not commodifiable in general. By contrast, I focus here on the cultural and organizational work involved in making the procurement and exchange of these goods socially acceptable and morally worthwhile.

My argument is in three parts. First, I draw an analogy between the problems faced by advocates of life insurance in the nineteenth century and advocates of organ procurement in the 1970s and '80s. Viviana Zelizer's work on the former provides a rich set of ideas with which to approach the latter.[3] Second, I discuss the efforts of donor families and transplant professionals to convince the public that organ donation is a worthwhile and appropriate act. I trace the development of their account of donation, and show how it has tended to rely on a particular set of arguments and stories. Third, I examine the growing importance of monetary incentives in organ procurement, and show how recently proposed systems of payment for organs recognize the expressive role of money. Throughout, I want to show how the exchange system in human organs is best understood as a carefully differentiated set of relationships rather than a simple yes-or-no answer to the question of commodification.

Reasons for Giving

Although the organ supply has grown steadily since the late 1980s, it has not kept pace with demand. As can be seen from figure 2.1, in 1988 just over four thousand cadaver donors were procured and there were about sixteen thousand people on the waiting list for a transplant. By 2004, the number of people waiting for transplants had risen to more than eighty thousand.[4] The number of cadaveric donors procured that year was just over seven thousand.[5] The shortfall is severe, and produces many tragic,

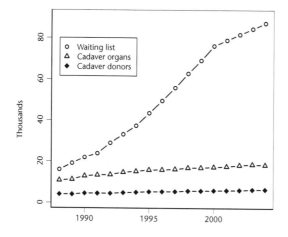

Figure 2.1. The extent of the cadaveric organ donor shortage: number of patients on transplant waiting lists and number of cadaveric donors and organs procured, 1988–2004

unusual, or otherwise vivid cases—a sick child waits for a new heart, a famous athlete gets a new liver, the family of a brain-dead accident victim refuses consent for organ procurement, and so on. One policy response to the shortfall is to introduce a financial incentive for the donation of organs—to create a production market for them. But to many commercial traffic in organs seems disturbing, even obscene. An altruistic system seems a more morally justifiable solution. The result has been a classic commodification debate. As I shall show, opposition to commodification can be traced in part to successful efforts to convince the public that organ donation is a morally worthwhile act. Public ambivalence about transplantation was overcome, in part, by arguing that donation was the "gift of life." The success of this idea now makes it more difficult to garner support for a market for organs.

With a few notable exceptions, sociologists have not paid much attention to organ transplants.[6] But we do know a good deal about how people think and talk about their own altruism, how they use money to express social ties, and how they manage money in personal relationships.[7] Research in this area suggests that the problem of commodification is not about the encroachment of the market on some untouched region of society. Rather, it is about the ways in which people account for their own actions and the place of money in their lives.

Take life insurance. As documented by Zelizer, life insurance was a controversial product in its early days and is a good example of moral debate about commodification. Though promoted by legislatures, life insurance companies were unsuccessful in the first half of the nineteenth century. Americans did not want to buy their product. This changed between 1840 and 1860, and insurance companies began to grow rapidly. By the late nineteenth century life insurance was commonplace, and the earlier controversy about it had abated.[8]

Life insurance was seen as threatening in that it assessed a person's life in financial terms. Compared to other examples of commodification, it now seems quite harmless. We would say that, unlike slavery, for example, it doesn't *really* put a cash value on you as a person. But many nineteenth century commentators felt it was just that: life insurance was "merchandising in human life" and "turning a very solemn thing into a mere commercial transaction." Americans did not want to buy life insurance because they did not want to put a price on their heads.[9]

There is also a close relationship between life insurance and death. A policy yields its reward when the owner dies, so buying life insurance meant tempting fate. Life insurers were aware of "the mysterious connection between insuring life and losing life," as customers confessed their fear that taking out a policy would hasten their deaths.[10] Such views are typical of the many traditional, magical strategies used to ward off death and illness (other examples include not mentioning death by name and not speaking the name of an illness for fear of contracting it). Social processes or professions related to death are usually subject to magic rituals of this kind. With life insurance, the presence of money required further ritual effort. The result was interesting. Death was not profaned by money. Rather, money could be transmuted into an offering of sorts, and life insurance made possible a proper, respectable—even lavish—funeral. Thus,

the dual relationship between money and death—actual as well as symbolic—is essential to the understanding of the development of life insurance. Sacrilegious because it equated cash with life, life insurance became on the other hand a legitimate vehicle for the symbolic use of money at the time of death.

In short, Zelizer argues, insurers had to reconcile the demands of business for profit with the sacred aspects of the good in question. One did not simply triumph over the other. Rather, contradictions were overcome through "the transformation of monetary evaluations of death into a ritual . . . life insurance assumed the role of a secular ritual that emphasized remembrance through money."[11]

Exchange in transplant organs raises similar issues, and it too provokes ritual responses. It introduces calculated medical decisions that not only are linked to death but must be made at the time of death by suddenly bereaved family members, face to face with their doctor in a hospital waiting room. The success of the entire national infrastructure of organ transplantation—its procurement organizations, monitoring systems, distribution networks, surgical teams, and so on—rests on how they understand the procurement process, and what they believe about it.

Organ procurement is done with great care, but it could hardly be more invasive. Donors are typically brain dead, their bodily functions mechanically sustained. The organs must be recovered as quickly as possible. In most cases, organ donation demands a remarkable sacrifice from someone who has just lost a close relative, usually through some violent accident. It is not obvious that people should consent to donation under these circumstances. Ruth Richardson has argued that the closest historical analog to organ harvesting is the dissection of the dead for anatomical study: "Both depend upon an accessible supply of dead bodies. Each damages the dead body for the sake of what is generally seen as a greater good. Both processes break cultural taboos."[12] Many religious doctrines pose potential stumbling blocks for donation. Some societies—Japan is the most prominent example—have opposed organ donation and transplants.[13] Even when generally accepted in a society, organ procurement can spark moral controversy.[14] In circumstances where there is a great shortage of organs—and the market seems like a possible solution to this problem—these difficulties are exacerbated. Over time, a cultural account of organ procurement, one that morally justifies and tries to motivate people to participate in it, has been built up.

We can trace how organ donation has been rationalized by OPOs and made meaningful by donor families. Zelizer describes three ways in which secular rituals developed around life insurance, in each case through the efforts of insurance providers and religious activists. First, it became a way for the bereaved to come to terms with the death of a loved one. Second, it became a moral act with religious significance. Third, it became a way to guarantee one's memory after death, and thus a kind of immortality. We can see a similar cultural account emerge in the mainstream media's discussions of organ transplantation, in the policy statements and promotional material of OPOs, and in published memoirs and other public discussions of transplantation.[15]

A Way to Cope with Bereavement

Between 1830 and 1870, life insurance companies justified their product as a way of coming to terms with death. Far more than a financial safety blanket, life insurance was a consolation "next to that of religion itself."[16]

In the first issue of the *American Life Assurance Magazine* (1860), Morris Franklin asserted that life insurance could "alleviate the pangs of the bereaved, cheer the heart of the widow and dry the orphan's tears." In a 1999 brochure, the United Network for Organ Sharing (UNOS) made the same argument about organ donation, albeit in less florid prose:

At the time of your death, your family will be asked about organ donation. Sharing your decision with your family will spare them the added burden of having to guess your wishes at a difficult time. . . . Carrying out your wish to save other lives can provide your family with great comfort in their time of grief.[17]

In most cases, donors become available for organ procurement through violent or accidental death.[18] The victims are often young, and their deaths are unexpected and meaningless. OPOs stress that organ donation can help a family make sense of such a tragedy and give some meaning to it. A number of journalistic and firsthand accounts from the point of view of donor families have been published. Their titles give a sense of their content: *Donor: How One Girl's Death Gave Life to Others, Lifeline: How One Night Changed Five Lives, The Nicholas Effect: A Boy's Gift to the World.*[19] In addition, organizations encourage donor families to tell their stories. It is not uncommon for these to be available online. (We have no comparable literature describing the experiences of those who refuse consent for organ donation, although we know that a substantial percentage of donation requests are refused.[20])

The online testimonies movingly articulate the grief of the families involved and relate their responses to the procurement request. They generally confirm the claims of OPOs that donating organs can invest an otherwise senseless death with some meaning. Alice Sanders is a typical example. She tells how she consented to have her husband's organs donated:

A day of sorrow for us turned into a very bright day for several families, as we were able to donate kidneys and the liver. My thought several times that day was how excited those recipients must have been when their pagers went off, knowing that they were getting a "second chance."[21]

In *The Nicholas Effect,* Reg Green describes how his seven-year-old son Nicholas was killed during a botched carjacking while the family was on holiday in Italy. His parents consented to donate their child's organs to the Italian procurement system. Seven Italians received Nicholas's organs.

The story provoked a tremendous response in Italy, resulting in, among other things, a jump in the donation rate there. This case brings out some subtle aspects of the gift relationship. Green's case provoked so much sympathy in Italy in part because a terrible thing happened while he was a visitor there. It seems fair to say the response might not have been as strong if the victim had been a local resident. While we normally care more for those closer to us, group identity can produce feelings of responsibility in circumstances like this. These feelings were amplified when Green acted so generously. As Mauss recognized, gift giving creates a bond of solidarity, as the giver shares what he has, but also a relationship of superiority, as he creates a debt that must be repaid.[22] The strong popular reaction can be seen as an expression of public feeling that the wrong done to him as a guest, combined with his selfless reaction to it, had created a debt that was almost impossible to discharge. The country was doubly in debt, shamed by a stranger's unwarranted generosity.[23]

The feelings expressed in the online memorials are much more varied and much less refined than those in the published books. Not all articulate the benefits of donation as well as Alice Sanders, or manage to find meaning in the way the Green family did. Some consist of a short note or poem expressing grief, nothing more. Sometimes writers express resentment at the anonymity of the donation procedure:

Oh, recipients where are you, you who live because our beloved donor has died? Can you not acknowledge your appreciation to your anonymous donor's beloved family? After all, the organ didn't come from a donor, it came from my beloved brother.[24]

Though the books too recount great suffering on the part of the families involved, they are positive and life-affirming. They can be read as "feeling rules."[25] They lay out a template for those who might be put in the same situation, following the story through to its moment of closure and acceptance. The narrative structure of the books aimed at adults follows the argument of the OPOs that donation helps families cope with death. As in the arguments for life insurance, the stress is on alleviating the "pangs of the bereaved." Though it is clear that not every donor family can follow it successfully, the books lay out a sequence, a set of stages of feeling centered on the benefits of organ donation in the face of an otherwise meaningless event.

This template for the secular ritual of organ donation is quite well established. The stock of cultural resources available to assist its broad acceptance is large (books, television documentaries, newspaper articles,

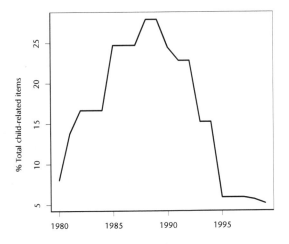

Figure 2.2. Percentage of *New York Times* stories about organ donation or transplantation mentioning infants or children, 1980–1999

and so on). The appearance of books aimed at children further indicate how entrenched this view now is. *Precious Gifts: Katie Coolican's Story* and *Lizzy Gets a New Liver* both lay out the process of organ and tissue donation for young children. *Precious Gifts* is aimed at four- to eight-year-olds. The publisher's description notes that the book will help "children and adults understand the process of organ and tissue donation. The determination of brain death and its meaning is clearly portrayed. The process of family decision-making is poignantly illustrated. A list of words and definitions is provided to enhance understanding."[26]

The place of children in this cultural account is interesting in another way, too. As organ donation became more common, media attention focused disproportionately on transplant cases involving infants or children. As can be seen from figure 2.2, *New York Times* coverage of child transplants rose and fell during the 1980s. Coverage spiked in 1984 with the story of Baby Fae, the "baby with the baboon heart," and remained high throughout the 1980s. Most of the stories late in the decade were about children getting transplants and (often) dying shortly afterward. By 1995, coverage of children fell to about 7 percent of total coverage and stayed there. The era of transplant "poster children" in the 1980s, however, may have done much to acquaint people with organ donation.

We might think it natural that organ donation should become a part of the process of mourning a family member lost in an accident. But in the early 1980s it was not clear to those involved whether a request for organs would make things better or worse for the grieving family. Writing in 1984, Arthur Caplan noted, "Most physicians and nurses do not want to inquire about organ donation. The highly emotional circumstances under which such requests are made make it uncomfortable for both families and medical personnel. . . . Moreover, at least some health professionals doubt that family members are able to give informed, voluntary consent in the context of the sudden death of a loved one."[27] Integrating organ donation into grieving required a good deal of cultural work. A combination of survey research conducted by the OPOs, widely circulated firsthand testimony from donor families, and required request laws that deprive nurses of discretion in the matter have essentially eliminated the idea (at least amongst transplant professionals) that a sympathetic request for organs could cause harm.[28]

A Moral Act for Family or Community

Religious leaders play an important role in making practices like organ donation acceptable. Church authorities in many religious traditions support organ donation. Their main concerns have been to assure that the donation is altruistic and that the donor is dead before the organs are removed. The accurate determination of death is important for theological reasons. In Catholic teaching, the soul must have left the body before organ harvesting can occur. Any move to redefine the moment of death is regarded with suspicion, as this might make it easier for doctors to give up on patients in order to harvest their organs.[29] But insofar as the donor is dead and there is no money involved, most Christian church authorities are not against organ donation.

Orthodox Judaism, however, has had more trouble assimilating organ donation to existing law and practice. There is more opposition to organ donation, and religious authority is more divided on the issue. Rabbis who favor it have had to make strong efforts to integrate organ donation into existing theology and ritual. Those in favor say, "The preservation of human life supersedes all *halachic* prohibitions, except for the three cardinal sins: idolatry, adultery and murder. Thus, procurement of cadaver organs for life-saving purposes need not pose a major problem, since the various prohibitions cited would be overridden by the supreme requirement to save a life."[30] A difficulty is that influential halachic opinion identifies the absence of a pulse as a necessary condition for determining death. This is almost never the case with organ donation, where the potential donor is brain dead but otherwise functioning.

While the dominant religions in the United States accept or encourage voluntary donation, these endorsements may go against the grain of other religious views on issues involving human goods and human life (such as genetic engineering and fetal research).[31] Support for organ donation in the Catholic church is weakened by concerns over the definition of brain death, which leads some conservative church members to oppose organ donation. When added to the difficulties within Judaism, it is not surprising that many people believe that religious officials oppose donation. A 1990 survey found that 61.5 percent of respondents believed that some major Western religions do not support it.[32] To combat these beliefs, UNOS and various individual OPOs collect and publicize official religious policies on organ donation and offer guidebooks to ministers on their role in the process.[33]

The success of these efforts can be gauged by looking back to the early reactions of religious authorities to organ transplants. In 1980, for example, Pope John Paul II expressed concern about a whole array of new medical technologies. He argued that the medical profession ought to consider "the implicit danger to man's right to life of such discoveries in the field of artificial insemination, birth and fertility control and hibernation, of retarded death, of genetic engineering, of the psychic drugs, of organ transplants."[34] He also suggested that the bodily "demolition and reconstruction" of transplant operations threatened the "psychological and physical integrity" of the patient. Throughout the 1980s, transplant advocates worked to detach organ transplants from issues like genetic engineering and fertility control, and argued strongly that both the life-saving nature of a transplant and the charitable act of donation were uncontroversial moral goods. They were largely successful in this, and although its early disquiet about transplants lingered in the public mind, the Catholic church itself never condemned transplantation and came to endorse it more enthusiastically, though always with the provisos that the organs always be gifts and that recipients not be used as a means to medical experimentation.[35]

For most Christian churches, the problem of organ transplants had to do with organ donation's proximity to death. Once church leaders had satisfied themselves that brain death was a valid concept, they no longer opposed organ donation. All major Christian denominations came to support donation and transplantation as a morally valuable activity. The other boundary problem—where human goods change hands for money—remained in the background, as there seemed to be little prospect of the legal sale of organs in any form.

A Way to Ensure One's Memory

The third feature of the cultural account of organ donation is the idea that donation is a way to live on (and do good) after death. Donor families, OPOs, and the media all express this sentiment. The "Donor Memorial Quilts" project (like the AIDS quilt) remembers the sacrifice of organ donors. A more direct expression of this idea is the notion that the donor spiritually as well as physically lives on in the recipient. Batten and Prottas's follow-up study of organ donor families found that 68 percent of them agreed that the deceased relative could live on in someone else through donation.[36] This sentiment is very common in the journalistic literature. OPOs also draw on it in their efforts to recruit people to sign organ donor cards.[37]

For example, the Sharing Network, a New Jersey OPO, organizes public information sessions where donor families and transplant recipients talk about their experiences. One participant, Jack Locicero, lost his daughter Amy in the 1993 Long Island Railroad shooting, when Colin Ferguson killed six people on a crowded commuter train. Locicero and his wife decided to donate Amy's organs. In a 1999 talk, he described how they came to meet some of the recipients, and how they had become "like family" to them since then.[38] The families feel that Amy lives on through her transplant. Kinlike ties have developed between them, especially between the Lociceros and the recipient of Amy's heart, a woman named Arlene. They visit one another. She sends flowers to Amy's mother on Mother's Day. When they first met, Arlene embraced Amy's mother and said, "The heart that beats in me once beat in your womb."

I highlight this case because, although such stories are common in the media, they are rare in practice. The Lociceros ended up meeting the recipients of their daughter's organs because of the publicity that the shooting received. *People* magazine picked up the story and traced the patients who had received the organs. Donor families are normally given the age, gender, and general location of each recipient. But much of the donor literature (though not the written OPO material) focuses on these unusual cases where families meet. The idea of the continuing life of the donor in the body of the transplant recipient is especially forceful in these cases. John Pekkanen describes one such meeting. One family member says, "I don't really see why we should have rules against these meetings. . . . I sure think it would help heal a lot of anger and hurt."[39]

The available evidence suggests that donor families are sometimes unhappy with the information they receive about the recipients of their gift.

In a valuable but unpublished pilot study, Maria Banevicius interviewed donor families about their experiences with donation. She found that all the families would have liked to receive some follow-up information about the recipient. One suggested a letter "maybe once a year. . . . I don't need to know every breath they take but you would like to know that they're okay or they're not okay."[40] Another respondent asked,

Wouldn't it be nice to be able to drop somebody a note, saying congratulations I'm glad everything went well for you. It was my relative who's [sic] part you received and I'm so glad to know you're no longer on dialysis, or that you can get up and go to work or go play tennis again. But there isn't that kind of an exchange, and why?[41]

These personal comments and the public account that goes with them are a clear manifestation of the Maussian idea that a gift is inalienable—that it bears the identity of the giver in a significant way. It might seem surprising to see this aspect of the gift relationship emphasized when organ donation is anonymous. Most donor families will not meet "their" organ recipients. The feeling that their loved one lives on must be more abstract.

Again, narrative accounts act as a road map for the emotions. They show how donors and donor families can form a meaningful sense of the continuing survival of the donor and a resulting emotional tie with recipients' families. This ideal must be promoted: it is not the only possible response. Evidence for the alternatives comes from both donors and recipients. Victoria Poole's *Thursday's Child* describes her son Sam's illness and eventual heart transplant. After his transplant, Sam reacts to his new heart like this: "My new heart likes me; I can feel it. Boy, am I glad I don't ever have to know where it came from or whose it was. I don't ever want to know. It's my heart now, and nobody is going to take it away from me"[42] This attitude is not found in the more recent literature.

On the donor family side, Banevicius found that although the families wanted more information, they were not always happy when they got it. In particular, four of her ten respondents were surprised and somewhat upset to find that "their" transplant recipient was not who they imagined. One said:

There was a 42 year-old man that had gotten the heart and in a way it was, which I now realize is silly, but it was almost a disappointment that it wasn't a 19 year-old girl. It could be because it would have been like my daughter was living again because, it would have been someone the same age she was.

And another:

I found it a little bit disconcerting that an 18 year-old heart went into such an—I don't want to say such an old person but it would be my hope that it would be someone younger, that would have 40 or 50 years left of their life. I don't want to say it was a waste, but I think that it would be more valuable maybe in somebody in their 20s.[43]

These reactions, on both sides, again point toward the active construction of a particular way of understanding the transplant process. Each element of the gift relationship—the moral obligation to give, the uniqueness or inalienability of what is given, the ties that the gift establishes between the parties—is found in the public account. The official version may diverge from the complex feelings of donor families and recipients. The dominant interpretation, as found in the Lociceros' experience and most of the book-length accounts, is perhaps the better, more satisfying one; it is not built in to the experience of donation, but the result of long-term efforts to make a complex medical procedure comprehensible in terms of the institution of gift giving.

The Expressive Role of Money

The National Organ Transplantation Act of 1984 prohibits organ sales. It was enacted partly in response to several reports of people trying to sell kidneys or corneas through the newspapers. The efforts of a Dr. H. Barry Jacobs provided a further spur. He planned to buy organs from around the world and sell them at a profit to those who needed them.[44] Public opposition to such schemes has remained high, despite the organ shortage, and politically the idea has long been thought untouchable.

Organ procurement is a delicate affair that must be handled with great sensitivity if it is to work at all. Those in favor of a purely altruistic system would say that this need for sensitivity and respect is one of the strongest arguments for keeping money and the market as far away from potential donors and their families as possible. They argue that a gift is the only form of exchange appropriate to such a situation. To offer cash for organs would be obscene. Their opponents retort that the real obscenity is a chronic shortage that could be solved by the market. Proposals for market solutions to the organ shortage have been gaining ground recently in the bioethics literature. In the introduction to their anthology on the subject, Arthur Caplan and Daniel Coelho note a shift toward arguments in favor of commodification: "Proposals for outright organ sales are suggested by authors who only years earlier had summarily dismissed any commodification of organs."[45]

This change in attitude seems to be driven in part by the increasing gap between the number of available transplant organs and the number of people who need one. Both in theory and in practice, bioethicists and the transplant community have begun to look for a way to increase the organ supply by using some financial incentive. Perhaps because the feeling rules for altruistic organ donation are now so well established—people know what organ donation is, what everyone's motives are, and how they ought to react—using money to reduce the shortage has become more plausible. The key to understanding the role of money in this area, I argue, lies in its expressive rather than its instrumental qualities. Rewards are set up so they are commensurable to the organ being exchanged; the payment reimburses the donor in an appropriate way.[46]

As noted above, the normative question—should organs be bought and sold?—tends to overwhelm the empirical one. From a sociological perspective, we should be interested in the practical solutions that emerge. I argue that we should expect money to play an expressive role in the exchange of organs. People make myriad efforts to arrange and earmark different transfers with tokens of payment so that they express the social relationship between the parties.[47] These efforts become especially creative in cases where a transaction involves something thought to be beyond the reach of utilitarian calculation.

If we look at proposals for organ sales, we find that this expressive aspect becomes more prominent the more practical the proposal is thought to be. Proposals for futures markets in organs try to eliminate the role of the donor family by making a contract with the donor. Early proposals that incorporated the donor family called for a cash bounty to be paid on receipt of the organs. This idea is no longer popular. Instead, those in favor of commodifying organs are careful to qualify what they mean. For instance, Blair and Kaserman, strong advocates of a market for organs, say,

> Because the issue of organ markets is so emotionally charged and often misunderstood, let us be clear about what is not being proposed. We do not propose barkers hawking human organs on street corners. We do not envision transplant patients, or their agents, dickering for a heart or liver with families of the recently deceased. We do not advocate an auction in which desperate recipients bid against each other for life-sustaining organs.

Instead, they propose offering potential suppliers "some fixed payment (either in cash or in the form of a tax credit) in exchange for entering into a binding contract that authorizes the removal of one or more of their organs at death."[48]

Why should they bother with this qualification? Such efforts to distinguish appropriate from inappropriate sales suggest that even market advocates are aware of the need to mark or transform the place of money in this context. The focus on appropriate tokens of payment is important. Certain exchanges are ruled out, especially cash payment at the point of sale. Instead, less visible payments are proposed, usually involving money given well in advance of any organ procurement. Even these payments may be further restricted to, for instance, a health insurance premium reduction.[49]

The futures market some propose would give buyers an *option* on an organ, should one become available.[50] Under such a system, most people's organs would not come up for donation, as they would not die in appropriate circumstances. In contrast to early schemes that proposed paying a donor's family as much as several thousand dollars (estimated prices varied widely), the amount of money on offer would be relatively small. In addition, the form of the payment would be commensurate with the item being purchased. The seller would receive a small annual reduction in health insurance costs—not a check, a holiday in the Bahamas, or a Wal-Mart gift voucher. The uncomfortable image of paying cold cash for a warm kidney is thus kept well away.

In practice, though, the decision to donate is made by the deceased person's family or next of kin. They are the real donors. Even if doctors know their patient wanted to donate his or her organs (and perhaps carried an organ donor card), hospital staff will almost always defer to the family's wishes. If they refuse consent, the organs will not be harvested. This is so even in cases where organ donor cards are witnessed legal documents. The central role of donor families is a big stumbling block to the implementation of payment schemes that involve making contracts with prospective donors before their deaths. More recent proposals have sought ways to reimburse donor families without paying them directly. In March 1999, state health officials in Pennsylvania announced that they would soon begin offering a three hundred–dollar stipend to help donor families cover funeral expenses. This was the first time that a definite amount of money had been introduced by an OPO in connection with donor families. Families were not to receive a cash payment, however: the payment was to be made to the funeral home. A spokesperson for the Gift of Life Program, the Delaware Valley's OPO, said at the time, "This is absolutely not buying and selling organs. . . . This is about having a voluntary death benefit for a family who gave a gift."[51] But of course, the OPO introduced the scheme in order to boost donation rates. ("The intent is to test it and see if it makes a difference to families," said the same spokesperson.) This is exactly how we would expect money to be introduced in such a case: it might be expected to act as an incentive, but it cannot be presented as one. Even this indirect method of payment proved too much for the Department of Health and Human Services, however, which replaced the funeral benefit with reimbursement for food and lodging expenses. The difficulty with this alternative is that organ procurement happens quickly, and donor families do not usually stay in a hotel (or go to a restaurant) during or just after making their decision.[52]

How market-based will exchange in organs become? At present, organs are given as gifts and for-profit exchange is illegal. However, media evidence shows that discussion of cash incentives for organs has consistently increased since the late 1980s. Figure 2.3 shows a smoothed plot of the number of *New York Times* news items mentioning financial incentives for organ donation, as a percentage of all stories about organ donation, over a twenty-year period. The jump in coverage around 1984 is caused by early reports about people trying to sell their kidneys, and by the subsequent passage of the National Organ Transplantation Act of 1984, which banned such sales. For the next several years, about 5 percent of all organ donation stories mentioned organ sales or financial incentives, but around 1990, the prevalence of market-related stories began to climb again. Later items tend to be policy-oriented discussions of financial incentives as a potential solution to the organ shortage, rather than news stories about organ sales.[53]

Commodification and Account Giving

The trend of public discussion documented in figure 2.3 and policy experiments like the Pennsylvania program suggest that money is being introduced to the act of donation in subtle ways. Does this mean organ procurement will ultimately be market-driven?

Some economists take this view. Their argument is that money is money. Proposals to provide payment in some other form or by some other name are just window dressing for the simple, rational expansion of the market into a new arena. The life insurance case shows that people often resist the market on moral grounds only to later accept it as expedient and sensible. Likewise for organ transplants. What would be the problem with an organ market? If it makes you feel better to call the sellers "donors" (as with human eggs), then go ahead. Whatever they are called, the suppliers will still get the market rate.

Work in economic sociology points in a different direction. Charles

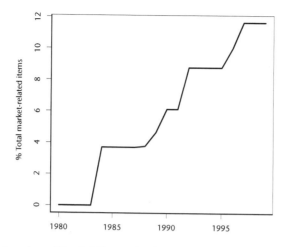

Figure 2.3. Percentage of *New York Times* stories about organ donation mentioning financial incentives for organ donation in their headline or lead paragraphs, 1980–1999

Tilly comments that, from Zelizer's perspective, "what appear to be narrowly rational economic transactions actually result from pursuit of meaningful social relations. Hence fears that monetization and commodification are dessicating social life have their causality backwards."[54] The efforts people make—the distinctions they draw, the categories they construct, the tokens they choose to pay with—are made because they mean something. These efforts express some underlying value or relationship that the alternatives would not capture properly. This something is sometimes difficult to specify. Margaret Radin, for instance, uses terms like "human flourishing" and "personhood" to try to grasp what would be lost if market rhetoric dictated our thoughts and actions.[55]

Is there evidence to help choose between these alternatives? Some cases do seem to favor one side than the other. Egg "donors" who are paid thousands of dollars for their services support the economistic view. On the other hand, the case of organ donation raises the question of why there should be so much window dressing in the first place. Why would people go to such enormous efforts to distinguish forms of payment and ritualize exchanges if their actions didn't express something besides a simple preference?

Even in the restricted area of human goods, there is a good deal of variation that does not conform to any simple pattern. Cash for organs is out of the question at present, but direct payment to women for their eggs is routine. Is the distinction therefore between renewable and nonrenewable body parts? This is a common explanation, but it is wrong. Except in special circumstances, whole blood cannot be bought from blood donors. In fact, a large cash-for-blood market in the United States was dismantled in the 1970s—a clear counterexample to the idea that market exchange must spread to everything in this area sooner or later.[56] This example should give pause to both sides. On the one hand, markets do not inevitably win out. There is no slippery slope toward commodification. But on the other, there is no fundamental fact about people that prevents for-profit markets in human goods from being set up. Just such a market existed for blood until 1974 and still exists for plasma. These are choices about how to value and exchange things, not immutable facts about human nature.

Further, the legitimate *expression* of a market interpretation might vary by social position or by the frequency of the transaction. Most donor families are only in that position once. Medical professionals who are repeatedly involved in organ exchange may have a more cynical view. "Backstage" cynicism is not uncommon in medicine. For instance, in the United Kingdom, when a person dies a doctor must fill in a form registering the cause of death. There is no charge to the next of kin for this. However, if the body is to be cremated, the doctor charges for the relevant form and gets another doctor to fill in a similar form, for a total charge of about sixty pounds. This is known in the trade as "ash cash." Even here, though, the market talk may represent rhetorical gallows humor more than a real financial incentive.[57]

Within genuinely cash-oriented markets, some interesting conventions still exist. Egg suppliers will normally receive an unspecified gift in addition to the money. The following newspaper advertisement (from the *Columbia Daily Spectator*) is typical: "Although our gratitude cannot be measured in dollars, if we were in your shoes, the least we would expect is: $6,500 plus expenses (and a gift)."[58] Even sperm donors, who are at the very bottom of the status and income hierarchies in the world of human goods, are still donors rather than vendors. It seems that, even if money is involved in these exchanges, people do not want to account for them in market terms. They repeatedly insist that they are not being motivated by the money.

Disguised payments, benefits, and gifts to donor families are likely to play an increasingly important role in the organ supply. Is this commodification? It does not conform to the altruistic vision of organ exchange. But neither it is the world of cash for kidneys that many opponents of commodification fear so much. Nor does it much resemble the system of binding contracts with future donors proposed by the more thoughtful advocates of the market. From what we know about the motives of donor families, the organizational effort required to procure organs, and the fragility of consent, there is every reason to believe that these complicated arrangements are a necessary part of motivating exchange, not just window dressing that could be dispensed with if only we were honest with ourselves.

———

Contemporary debate about medical technology and the market is attracted by novelty, by the brave new worlds opened up by genetic engineering or cloning or xenotransplantation.[59] It is often normative, asking what ought to be done (to commodify or not to commodify) with particular goods.[60] These are important problems, but I have taken a different tack here. I argue that economic and cultural sociology contribute important insights about how people manage these problems. This approach, developed from historical cases of commodification, makes good empirical predictions about the organ industry. I argue that the chief lesson of these studies is that the empirical reality of organ exchange is likely to be more differentiated and carefully managed than standard debates about commodification might lead us to believe.

Though outside the range of the usual comparison cases, the analogy between the life insurance and organ transplant industries is rich. Life insurance and organ transplants threaten sacred beliefs about death and the body, bringing with them the threat of utilitarian calculation and the negative influence of money. One possible reaction is to ban the corrupting practice for good. But more often the practical benefits are large, or the promoting organizations are powerful. The new practice can be reinterpreted in a way that allows it to be incorporated into existing ritual and reconciled to existing understandings. The cultural account of organ donation can been seen in these terms. Transplant advocates did not force their ideas on an unwilling public. Neither did the account of donation appear by magic to solve the problem of procurement. Rather, there are many ways that donation might be understood. The cultural work of transplant advocates produced the public version we ended up with. They found ways to incorporate donation into death rituals; they made signing a donor card a morally worthwhile action; they associated the donation with a kind of social immortality. The result is that public opposition to organ procurement is now almost unknown in the United States, even though people do not like to sign donor cards, families often refuse consent to donate, and the available evidence suggests a much wider range of responses to procurement than does the official account.

As the organ shortage has worsened, OPOs have begun to explore new ways to give people incentives to donate. Proposals for commercializing the system by contracting with potential donors misunderstand both how the procurement process works and how people understand it. Paradoxically, opposition to commercialization is buttressed by the same arguments for the "gift of life" that helped legitimate donation and transplantation from the 1970s onward. In response, transplant advocates in favor of some kind of incentive system are beginning to develop payment systems that reimburse without corrupting. A new phase of account making seems to be under way.

The standard commodification literature tends to miss this organizational and cultural work. Instead, it focuses on abstract questions of commodification or on difficult (and often quite unusual) cases.[61] Some bioethicists are explicitly concerned with the practical application of moral theory, but the field as a whole has little to say about the ways individuals and organizations have found ways to give meaning to transplantation.[62] Similarly, although some scholars have developed sophisticated conceptual accounts of commodification they have less to say about the organizational effort and cultural work that go into making these exchanges socially acceptable.[63]

Like those in similar areas that deal with death or the exchange of human goods, the transplant community has tried to account for itself as a moral actor in a comprehensible and convincing way. In the process it has developed a body of secular ritual to help manage a fragile transaction. This account is under increasing pressure as the gap between supply and demand for organs continues to widen. The key to understanding what exchange in human goods will look like in the future does not lie in novel technologies or moral recipes. Rather, what is important is its resemblance to other markets—for insurance, care, children, or sex—that are subject to similar cultural work and face comparable organizational problems. Strategies used to make exchanges socially acceptable in these cases will also shape the institutionalization of organ donation.

THREE

The Logistics of Altruism

New treatments are developed all the time in medicine, and many of them end up becoming routine options for care. Most involve a new surgical procedure or drug that, once tested and perfected, can be made widely available in a short time. Organ transplants are different. Surgical techniques pioneered in the 1970s and immunosuppressive drugs developed in the 1980s have made them widely available, but transplants cannot happen without a reliable supply of fresh human organs. As we saw in chapter 2, these are in very short supply. At present they come almost entirely from two sources: *Cadaveric donors* are brain-dead individuals whose bodies are kept functioning artificially. Their families or next of kin consent to the organ harvesting. *Living donors* are usually related by blood or marriage to the transplant recipient. Of the twenty-seven thousand organs transplanted in the United States in 2004, 74 percent came from cadaveric donors and the remainder from living donors.

Because of the shortage of organs, convincing people to become donors has always been at the center of the cultural account of organ donation. We saw in chapter 2 how this account took shape in the media's coverage of organ donation, in popular books about it, and in the policy statements and publicity materials of the United Network for Organ Sharing and its organ procurement organizations. The result of this process, I argued, was a consensus that organ donation was a good thing ethically and medically. There is no longer much public controversy about the morality of organ donation or procurement. However, as we shall see, this consensus does not mean that ordinary people are always prepared to donate their organs or those of their loved ones. Obtaining consent from donor families remains more difficult than the widespread support for donation would lead one to expect. OPOs therefore face a twofold challenge. They must solve the technical problems of finding, preserving, and transporting suitable organs, and they must convince grieving families to say yes to donation.

These problems are severe. There is a gulf between the image of the altruistic individual volunteering her organs and the enormous logistical efforts of OPOs to secure donors. This chapter turns away from the cultural account of donation to examine the large-scale structure of exchange in organs in the United States. The central question is simple: Why do some OPOs procure more donors than others? I will argue that focusing on the organizational basis of procurement goes a long way toward answering this question. Beyond the immediate empirical question, I argue that the widespread emphasis on the altruism of individual donors distracts us from the remarkable organizational achievement that the procurement system represents, and from the essentially structural problems that it faces. The ongoing debate over whether organ procurement should be commodified pays little attention to the complex, rationalized system of procurement and exchange that already exists. We can say that the donor procurement system helps produce altruism through its policies, practices, and cultural work and that it has *industrialized* altruism by treating it as a resource-extraction problem.

Some OPOs procure more donors than others. What is it about these organizations or their environments that makes them better or worse at what they do? To answer this question, I analyze the pattern of procurement rates in the United States in 1997. This kind of analysis poses several challenges. Previous efforts to compare procurement rates, for example, have usually relied on data for aggregate regions and not particular OPOs. When organizations rather than regions have been studied, procurement rates have not always been measured accurately, or only a small number of organizations have been analyzed. Information about the varying policies of OPOs exists, but it has not been linked to procurement rates. This chapter brings together accurate data about procurement rates, organizational structure, policies, and the environmental characteristics of OPOs in an effort to understand why rates of organ donation vary across the country. I begin with a description of how OPOs are organized and how the current system developed.

The Public's Reluctance to Donate

Until about 1980, successful organ transplants were rare. Although reliable surgical techniques to transplant most major organs were available by the 1970s, preventing patients' immune systems from rejecting the new organs proved difficult. Most patients died of complications arising from rejection. In the early 1980s, a new generation of immunosuppressive therapies was introduced. These therapies reduced the chances that a recipient's immune system would reject the transplanted organ. The success of cyclosporine and other such drugs led to a rapid increase in the number of transplants in the United States. There are now more than twenty-seven thousand organ transplants performed every year in the United States. The majority of these (16,000) are kidney transplants, with livers (5,800), hearts (2,000), and lungs and pancreases (about 1,000 each) making up most of the rest of the total.

As transplants became more successful, transplant organs rapidly became scarce. Demand for organs now greatly outruns their supply (see fig. 2.1). To meet this demand, a network of organ procurement organizations collects and distributes organs from donors. This is a difficult task. Although the number of transplants doubled between 1988 and 2004, the number of donors rose at a slower rate. On average, about three organs are now harvested from every donor. Many more parts—heart valves, skin, cartilage, and so on—can be obtained if conditions are right. At one time, transplant programs were less common and some kinds of transplant surgery were still being developed. This meant that many organs from a particular donor might go unused. Over time, more kinds of transplants have become possible and surgeons have become more adept at performing them, so few viable organs from an available donor now go to waste. A good portion of the increase in the number of transplants is thus attributable to improvements in the efficiency of transplant surgery and the greater variety of transplants that can be routinely carried out. The rate of cadaveric procurement has, since 1988, risen at an average annual rate of just over 3 percent, with considerable year-to-year and regional variation. At the same time, though, living donors have become an important source of organs, especially kidneys. The majority of transplanted kidneys now come from living donors.[1]

As we saw in the previous two chapters, organ donation has the potential to be controversial. Outside of the United States, comparative evidence shows that organ donation is often viewed with suspicion or even hostility.[2] By contrast, public opinion polls suggest that Americans are broadly in favor of organ donation. In a 1993 Gallup poll conducted for a

Boston OPO, 85 percent of respondents said they supported organ donation in general, with 6 percent opposing it and 9 percent saying they didn't know. Surveys consistently find, however, that support for donation is significantly lower among nonwhite respondents. Only 75 percent of Hispanic and 69 percent of black respondents were generally in favor of donation, in contrast to 87 percent of whites.[3]

Beyond general expressions of support for donation, things are rather more mixed. Only 37 percent say they are "very likely" to have their organs donated after their death; about the same number say they have told their family members that they do not want to become organ donors. Money complicates the situation further. Although many transplant advocates are convinced that for-profit organ donation would be a disaster (and the cultural account of donation focuses exclusively on altruistic donation), opinion poll data suggests that people are more ambivalent. In the same Gallup poll, 81 percent of respondents said that a financial incentive would have no effect on their likelihood of donating a family member's organs. Only 5 percent said it would make them less likely to donate, and 12 percent said it would make donation more likely. The 1996 General Social Survey probed a little more deeply into this issue. The survey asked respondents, "Should a person be allowed to sell their kidney to a hospital or organ center?" and also "What is the best way to allocate organs for transplant?" The answers were sharply divergent. Although 36 percent thought that one should definitely not be allowed to sell a kidney, 17 percent said "probably yes" and 19 percent "definitely yes." On the question of who should receive transplant organs, respondents were given a choice between several allocation methods: lottery, auction, merit (the criteria were left unspecified), and first come, first served. Despite the wide range of opinion on the right to sell an organ—and the fact that 36 percent of respondents expressed moderate or strong support for the idea—only about 1 percent thought that organs would be best allocated by auction. More than 81 percent favored "first come, first served."[4]

Although most Americans express support for organ donation, far fewer are prepared to take the steps necessary to becoming an organ donor (signing a donor card, discussing it with their families, and so on). Further, their ideas about the proper role of money and the market are mixed. When asked if they should be allowed to sell their own organs, many will assert some kind of right to do so. But when asked about allocation (and thus put in the position of someone needing an organ) the great majority would prefer to form a line and wait, rather than have to rely on money. As the argument in chapter 2 suggests, public resistance to organ markets seems to come in large part from a combination of the structure of the potential market and the form of the payment. Hence auction-type markets, which suggest frantic competition with the goods always going to the wealthiest bidder, get a very negative reaction. But this does not extend to an outright rejection of markets in human goods.

How Organ Procurement Is Organized

When it comes to procurement, we must shift our attention away from the vagaries of public opinion. We need instead to understand the organizations that collect and distribute the organs. The OPO network is where abstract concepts like altruism, donation, ownership, and commodification become hard logistical problems.

The question of who owned transplant organs was never really asked in the United States until the mid-1980s, when the transplant industry began to expand rapidly. Through the 1960s and 1970s, it was taken for granted that human organs belonged to the surgeons who had removed them from donors, and these surgeons decided who received organs for transplant, on the basis of whatever ethical and clinical criteria they saw fit to apply. There was a good deal of consistency, because transplant surgeons were all members of the same profession, had been through more or less the same kinds of training, and had adopted more or less similar values. But there were no formal regulations. Individual surgeons were accountable to themselves and perhaps to colleagues in their transplant centers. Organs were obtained, distributed, and transplanted locally. The rule was, in effect, "Every surgeon a king, and every city a kingdom."[5]

The two dominant features of this old system were, first, that the organ, when it was exchanged, was allocated to the hospital and not the patient and, second, that whatever rules hospitals had for allocating organs were usually informal and unwritten. Surgeons drew on personal networks to allocate spare organs or search for suitable ones. Hospitals sometimes delegated allocation decisions to so-called God Squads, standing committees that decided who got available organs, sometimes using vague and potentially controversial criteria such as "contribution to the community."

The "cyclosporine revolution" of the early 1980s introduced new drugs that prevented transplanted organs from being immediately rejected by the immune systems of their recipients. This made successful transplantation possible on a much wider scale. It also made the old procurement and allocation system untenable. The government overhauled it in 1984 when it passed the National Organ Transplantation Act. Under this law, human organs must be given as gifts in the United States. Organs are a public good belonging to the state and cannot be sold. In theory, the deceased has the first and deciding voice about whether to donate them. If she has signed an organ donor card, then the organs may be removed. If not, the decision is made by someone else. There is a chain of priority, from spouses to parents to kin. If none of those can be found, the medical examiner decides. As was noted in chapter 2, however, this aspect of the law is most often ignored. Carrying a donor card is almost never a sufficient cause for removing organs if any family members are present. The next of kin is usually given the choice, and doctors will accept a decision not to give up the organs, even if it is known that the deceased wished to be a donor.[6]

The National Organ Transplantation Act also charged a task force with working out what the new procurement and allocation system should look like. The Organ Procurement and Transplantation Network was established under the aegis of the Department of Health and Human Services. Health and Human Services did not run the network, however. Instead, the contract to administer OPTN was put out for bids and awarded in 1986 to the United Network for Organ Sharing, a private, nonprofit corporation. Since 1977, UNOS had operated a regional donor registry as a branch of the South Eastern Regional Organ Procurement Foundation. It incorporated itself in 1984 in anticipation of the emergence of a national allocation system. UNOS has won the OPTN contract each time it has come up for renewal and at present has no plausible competitor for the job. Besides the organ procurement organizations, the other two main components of the transplant industry are 59 independent histocompatibility laboratories and 256 hospital transplant centers; all are members of UNOS. The labs carry out the tests that allow patients to be matched with compatible organs. The transplant centers are, of course, where the surgery actually happens.

UNOS allocates organs not nationally but by region (for administrative purposes, it divides the country into eleven regions, as shown in figure 3.1A). When UNOS took over the system in 1986, it was given power to set whatever allocation criteria it wanted. Its database allows it to match patients to organs first on the basis of more or less well-defined medical criteria, and subsequently by proximity. In 1997, there were sixty-one organ procurement organizations operating in the United States. Each one has the resources to procure, store, and deliver organs to transplant centers, where patients register on waiting lists. But there is considerable variation in procurement rates between these organizations. Figure 3.1B shows the boundaries of these OPOs. Borders are drawn at the county level and may cross state lines. In addition, some OPOs administer noncontiguous areas.

Some OPOs procure more donors than others, and some transplant

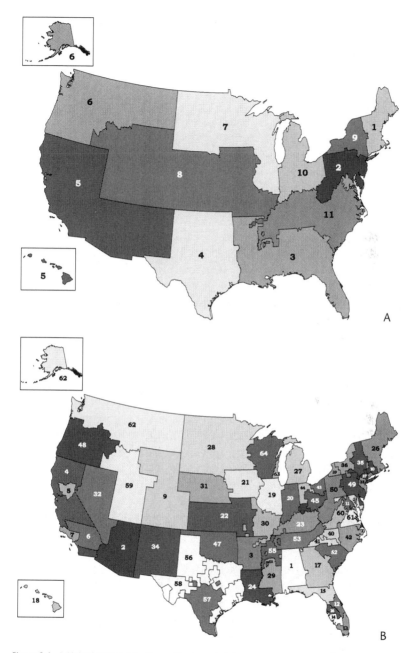

Figure 3.1. *A,* United Network for Organ Sharing administrative regions; *B,* Organ procurement organization boundaries in 1997

Note: The network is organized by county, with OPO boundaries often crossing state lines.

centers perform more operations than others. This means that the UNOS regions differ substantially both in the number of patients on waiting lists at centers within the region and in the mean wait time for a transplant. In 1997 patients in the southeast of the country waited about 180 days for a liver transplant, whereas patients in New England waited on average more than three years.

From about 1994 on, these disparities in wait times were the central issue in a long-running political controversy. The Department of Health and Human Services has repeatedly tried to change the allocation rules so that organs would be shared primarily on a national rather than a regional basis—if an organ became available, it would go to the sickest suitable person in the country, not necessarily someone in the region. This proposal, known as the DHHS "Final Rule," would mainly have affected the allocation of livers. It was generally accepted that changing the allocation system in this way would result in more organs going to a small number of big transplant centers, which tend to have many more seriously ill patients on their books. Without first claim on organs from their region, centers that carried out relatively few transplants per year would find it more difficult to do any procedures at all and might well be driven out of business.[7] According to UNOS, in August 1998 there were 124 liver transplantation programs in the United States, 26 of which had performed five or fewer transplants in the previous year.

UNOS consistently opposed the proposed changes, and the struggle between it and the DHHS became increasingly politicized. Between 1996 and 1999, Congress postponed the final implementation of the new allocation rules on a number of occasions, calling for more consultation time and more research. An independent report recommended in 1999 that the DHHS proposals be implemented, but Congress again postponed a decision until March 2000.[8] In the meantime, a number of states—typically those with an above-average donor yield, a below-average waiting-list time, or both—sought to make the limits of altruism coincide with the borders of the state. They passed "local-first" laws, specifying that organs donated within the state could be shipped outside it only if a suitable in-state recipient could not be found. Once the criterion of medical urgency is relaxed, of course, a suitable recipient can almost always be found. Louisiana, Oklahoma, Wisconsin, South Carolina, and Kentucky all passed laws of this kind. Local-first laws obviously go against the spirit of the National Organ Transplantation Act, which defines donated organs as a national good. While no one has yet suggested that people should only be eligible to list for transplants in the states they were born or live in, neither the ideals of citizenship nor the idea of a national community prevented these states from trying to restrict interstate commerce in this valuable resource. Moreover, the state of Wisconsin, together with a number of clinics and hospitals from other parts of the country, brought a lawsuit against the federal government, claiming that the proposed DHHS rule was an illegal extension of the department secretary's authority.[9]

In September 2000, after extensive negotiations, DHHS renewed UNOS's contract to run the Organ Procurement and Transplantation Network. The right to run the Scientific Registry of Transplant Recipients was, however, awarded to the University Renal Research and Education Association, a research body based at the University of Michigan. The registry is responsible for most of the data analysis of transplant records. Besides losing control of the Scientific Registry, for the first time since the late 1980s UNOS had competition for the contract to run the OPTN. The Center for Support of the Transplant Community, a new body based in Pittsburgh, put in a bid. This organization, which supported the DHHS final rule, was made up primarily of representatives of the larger transplant centers. (The University of Pittsburgh Hospital has the largest liver transplant program in the world.) Following his election, President George W. Bush appointed Tommy Thompson as secretary of Health and Human Services. Thompson is the former governor of Wisconsin and initiated both his state's local-first law and its case against the government department he then came to head.

These struggles have mainly been over the fairest way to allocate the scarce resource of organs for transplant. As a result, the organizational structure and politics of the organ procurement system have been brought into the spotlight in a way that had not happened before. Rather than praising or questioning the actions of heroic surgeons, as was more common in the pioneering days of transplantation, attention has focused on the business of procurement. It is clear from this battle just how valuable cadaveric donors are to OPOs and transplant centers, and how ambivalent many of them are about giving up the organs they procure to a nationwide mechanism of allocation. I will now construct a picture of the macrostructure of this exchange network and the procurement rates that underpin it.

Like any good that people or organizations trade among themselves, when viewed in the aggregate, exchange in human organs is a dynamic system. As soon as new organs are harvested, they enter into a national trade network and move across the country in response to a complex set of rules and conventions. An organ procured from an accident victim in Ohio, for instance, may turn out to be a perfect match for a patient at a center in Delaware. Some parts of the country do not have transplant centers; a few have large facilities that can accommodate many more patients than they have organs for. Some regions may find themselves with more organs than they can use at a particular moment.

Data on organ "trade flows" within the United States are not secret, but neither are they available in the same way as, for example, information about the interstate flow of money. Organ exchange is not part of the formal economy, even though organ transplants are expensive, hundreds of organs crisscross the country each day, and thousands of people queue up to wait for one. Inter-OPO exchange in kidneys is a partial exception. Almost all kidney transplants are funded by Medicare. To be reimbursed by the government for their services, OPOs must submit annual cost reports detailing, among other things, the number of kidneys they procured, how many were exported to other service areas, how many they imported, and how much the organs cost to process. Using this information, we can map the pattern of exchange in kidneys between OPOs.

This map is not an ideal representation of exchange in kidneys. Apart from being a static snapshot of a dynamic system, its main limitation is that it is not based on proper trade-flow data. We know only how many kidneys each OPO exported and how many it imported, not the origins of the imports or the destinations of the exports. If we subtract the number of kidneys that an OPO imported from the number it exported, we get its balance of trade. As with any good, net exporters can be said to run a surplus, while net importers run a deficit. The data for 1997 are mapped in figure 3.2.

A number of patterns are evident from this map. Most OPOs have a reasonably even balance of trade or a moderate deficit. Sparsely populated areas, which tend to procure fewer donors, also have fewer patients awaiting transplants. Thus the Pacific Northwest, Wyoming, Colorado, and New Mexico all have net balances close to zero. A smaller number of centers run large surpluses or deficits. There are more large exporters than large importers, and in most cases a large net importer will be located near more than one major exporter. There are four main centers of exchange. A band of high-export OPOs runs from Michigan south through Indiana into Kentucky and Tennessee. Just east of these OPOs is the area of western Pennsylvania and West Virginia administered by the Center for Organ Recovery and Transplantation. This OPO, the second largest importer of kidneys in the United States, is affiliated with the University of Pittsburgh Hospital, one of the largest transplant centers in the world. A second concentration of exchange is located in Texas. One OPO there, the Southwest Transplant Alliance, manages procurement in all of the state's major cities. Another, the Life Gift Organ Donation Center, is a major importer. In the Northeast, OPOs in New England, New York, and northern New Jersey are

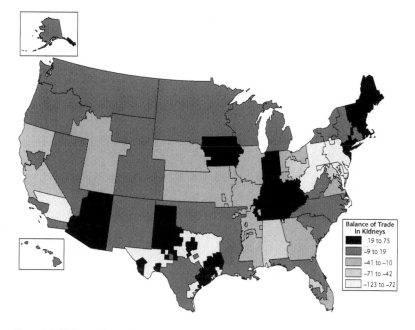

Figure 3.2. "Balance of trade" in kidneys, 1997
Note: Units are the raw number of kidneys exchanged between OPOs.

all strong net exporters, most likely to the cluster of transplant centers around Philadelphia, Delaware, and Washington, DC. On the west coast, the only major exporter is Golden State Donor Services (centered on Sacramento). Regional OPA of Southern California, which serves Los Angeles and Santa Barbara, is a small net exporter. Its neighboring OPO, which serves Orange County (and three others in the southern California desert), is the biggest importer of kidneys in the country. The OPOs just east of California (in Arizona, Nevada, and Utah) tend to have low donor yields and few transplant centers. They are net exporters. In general, then, the map shows the exchange network to be strongly regionalized and highlights the location of larger transplant centers that perform a disproportionate number of operations.

Explaining Variation in Procurement

With this more detailed picture of the structure of the national procurement system, and a good sense of how organs are exchanged across it, we can ask about the raw materials that make the exchange system possible in the first place. A better understanding of variation in procurement rates at the organizational level would cast light on the specific policy conflicts over allocation that were discussed above, as well as the more general question of how altruism is socially produced. Mapping procurement rates reveals suggestive geographical patterns, with OPOs in some areas of the country having much higher rates than others. We can also ask what predicts these patterns—are they wholly due to differences in the populations served by OPOs, or do some characteristics of the organizations themselves make a difference? Below, I present an analysis of procurement rates at the OPO level, incorporating measures of the structural and ecological characteristics of each service area and of the OPO's organizational structure and policies.

First, however, we need to know what we are measuring. The proper estimation of the procurement rate poses practical and political problems. To measure it for an OPO in a given year, we need to know the number of organs it actually procured and the number of cadavers from which organs could have been successfully harvested. The first quantity is known with certainty for every OPO in the country. The second is more difficult to estimate.

It is relatively easy to calculate the procurement rate per million population. The main advantage to measuring the procurement rate this way is that population data is available in detail and over time. But using population as the denominator when calculating a procurement rate is unsatisfactory. For one thing, the number represents the people in an OPO's catchment area who are alive, and ipso facto not candidates for organ harvesting. Nevertheless, performance measures for OPOs are often denominated in donors per million population. Federal rules require that an OPO be within 75 percent of the average rate on a number of performance measures, including procurement per million population, if it is to retain its certification. The OPOs have argued that efforts to compare organizations using this metric are misguided, because of the different populations they work with and the unpredictable way in which potential donors become available. This is not an unreasonable claim. Potential donors are usually victims of some kind of violent accident. Not every means of violent death yields a potential donor, but if the victim dies in a way that leaves most major organs intact then procurement may be possible. Even then, OPOs must overcome tight time pressures and other organizational challenges before a donor can be successfully procured.

As a further complication, different parts of the country, and hence different OPOs, are more or less likely to experience the kinds of events that

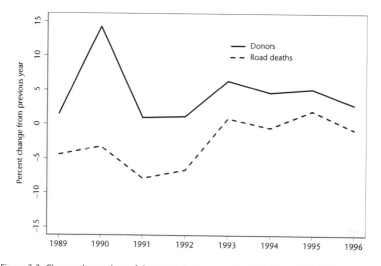

Figure 3.3. Changes in numbers of donors and of road accident fatalities, 1989–1996

produce potential donors. For example, motor vehicle accidents routinely account for a significant proportion of organ donors—a little more than a quarter in 1997. Parts of the country with high rates of road fatalities are more likely to yield a higher number of potential donors. Transplant professionals in New York recently lamented the state's continuously improving road safety record, which has cut back on the supply of donors. But the relationship between road safety and donation is not a simple one. Southern states have the highest road fatality rates, but their OPOs do not procure the most donors. This is because converting an accident victim into a donor also depends on a number of organizational factors that (as we shall see below) vary between OPOs. Across the country as a whole, donor procurement rates rose steadily during the 1990s, while road death rates declined over the same period. The two trends are strongly related, as can be seen in figure 3.3. This figure plots the rate of change in the procurement and road accident fatality rates from 1989 through 1996. As can been seen, the rate of change in number of donors is consistently positive, whereas the rate of change in road fatalities is generally negative. But the trend lines track each other closely from year to year, indicating that the rate of organ procurement is sensitive to changes in the road fatality rate, though the former is generally growing and the latter falling. As might be expected, the rate of change in organ procurement seems more volatile than the rate of change in road fatalities.

If we want to study the role of logistical and organizational factors in procurement, it is best to take these proximate causes of death out of the analysis altogether. We can do this by controlling for them in our measure of the procurement rate. A study by the General Accounting Office explored various measures.[10] Rather than using the live population as the denominator, they first suggested using the number of deaths for a given year. This is more accurate but still not entirely satisfactory. As we have noted, some people die in ways that rule out the use of their organs for transplant.[11] The GAO went on to recommend an adjusted death rate based on ICD-9-CM codes. These are codes specified in the International Classification of Diseases, Ninth Revision—Clinical Modification and used to classify deaths by cause and circumstances. Medical staff apply these codes at the time of death, and they are collected and reported nationally by the Centers for Disease Control and Prevention. Doctors can say with some confidence which causes of death would make procurement a realistic possibility in normal circumstances. This is still not quite a perfect measure, because ICD-9-CM codes do not always give enough information to say for certain whether a case involved a donor candidate or not. But it is a more focused measure than the raw death rate, and of course it is much better than any population-based estimator. This adjusted death rate is the best practical denominator for calculating the procurement rate, short of conducting a complete medical records review of every in-hospital death in every hospital in the United States over the course of a year—a course of action the GAO felt would be too difficult and costly even for the federal government.

As it happened, the GAO found that most OPOs ranked similarly in terms of efficiency under each of the three measures.[12] The stricter the measure became the more OPOs missed the mandated cutoff, but OPOs that missed on a less strict measure also missed on a more strict one. This suggests that the various denominators (live population, number of deaths, and adjusted number of deaths) represented the same underlying variable ("number of potential donors") with increasing accuracy.[13]

Figure 3.4 maps procurement rates by OPO for 1997. They vary from 16.4 to just over 70 donors per thousand evaluable deaths, with a median score of 42.5. There are some striking geographical patterns. The three highest-scoring OPOs—Life Source of the Upper Midwest, which procures from Minnesota and the Dakotas, and Wisconsin's two OPOs—are all in the upper Midwest. (Procurement organizations in Ohio, Iowa, and Nebraska are also in the top quartile; Michigan and Indiana lag behind their neighbors.) The Northeast also shows up strongly as a region with above-average procurement rates, though not as high as those in the upper Midwest. Elsewhere things are more variable. Some OPOs in Florida and Vir-

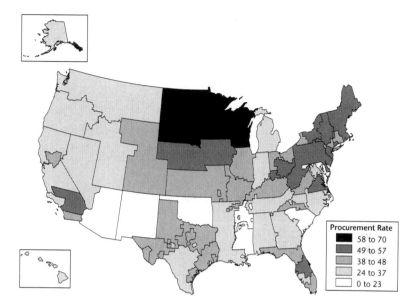

Figure 3.4. OPO donor procurement per thousand evaluable deaths, 1997

ginia rank highly. On the west coast, however, only the Southern California Organ Procurement Center performs well above average. (Recall that it is also the largest importer of kidneys in the country.) The Pacific Northwest, the Rocky Mountain states, California, and the Southwest are below average, in many cases far below. New Mexico, Arizona, Mississippi, South Carolina, and Maryland do worst.

Altruism as an Organizational Problem

In everyday usage, an altruistic act is one motivated by concern or regard for others rather than oneself. Roberta Simmons, a sociologist, gives a useful first definition: "Although scholars' definitions differ, most would agree that altruism (1) seeks to increase another's welfare, not one's own; (2) is voluntary; (3) is intentional, meant to help someone else; and (4) expects no external reward."[14] Elliot Sober and David Sloan Wilson (a philosopher and a biologist, respectively) observe, "The altruism hypothesis maintains that people sometimes care about the welfare of others as an end in itself. Altruists have irreducible other-directed ends."[15]

Explanations of altruism come in two broad varieties.[16] From an evolutionary perspective, altruism is a behavioral trait to be evaluated in terms of its effect on the reproductive fitness of altruistic agents. As Sober and Wilson put it, "Evolutionary biologists define altruism entirely in terms of survival and reproduction. A behavior is altruistic when it increases the fitness of others and decreases the fitness of the actor."[17] The problem, then, is to say how a behavior that helps others at a cost to oneself could have evolved. From a social-psychological perspective, altruism is a disposition or identity. The question here concerns purity of motive—whether people truly are altruistic, or whether their actions are covertly by selfish in some way.

Operational definitions of altruism are "theory-laden" in the sense that different research programs may have quite different goals in mind, and concepts of altruism are often tied to these programs. Evolutionary definitions require a net cost to the giver, but social-psychological definitions need not. This means there can be reasonable disagreement over how to classify possibly ambiguous actions like blood and organ donation, gifts to charity, volunteering, and so on. A direct conflict arises only where a theory insists that ostensibly well-intentioned actions must be selfishness in disguise. In his simplest form, for example, *Homo economicus* is both rational and wholly self-regarding, so he is incapable *ex hypothesi* of costly altruism. His apparently altruistic acts confer some kind of benefit on himself—either tangibly or in the form of a "warm glow." It is important to see that this view of altruism arises out of the constraints of a particular model of action rather than basic facts about the world. More sophisticated rational-choice models need not insist on this point and can make room for altruism in the common sense of the word. As David Schmidtz argues:

> It would be a mistake to say something cannot be altruistic if you really enjoy doing it. This would put the cart before the horse. If you help other people for their sake, you are altruistic whether or not you like having the concern for others that your action expresses. . . . Enjoying an action can affect its moral worth without changing the fact that it is altruistic.[18]

Schmidtz shows that reflectively rational agents (that is, agents who think about the effects of their choices on their preferences) can have reasons to cultivate an altruistic regard for others in the ordinary sense. Having a reason for doing something for someone—even a reason from one's own point of view—does not disqualify it from counting as altruistic.

In the evolutionary approach, altruism is treated as (or as if it were) a heritable trait. Research formally analyzes or numerically simulates the reproductive fitness of agents who behave altruistically toward other agents.

To count as such, altruists must help other (possibly selfish) agents at some cost to themselves and this behavior must then be selected for over time. This sort of altruism can evolve by way of biological or cultural mechanisms.[19] The rich body of work that analyzes this problem examines fundamental questions about the possibility of altruism in a very general way. It has less to say about the social organization of altruism in society, particularly the widespread and variable world of voluntary donation of the kind this book is about.

The social-psychological approach does focus on cases of deliberate altruism in human beings. Whereas the biological approach does not need a theory of intentions or motives to work, it is hard to ignore these when dealing with people. In fact, the goal is to develop a theory of these motives and the identities that generate them. Here again we find strong evidence that altruism is a common and stable phenomenon. Many people do act out of a regard for the well-being of others. They do not do so all the time, of course, but in many cases there is no good reason to suspect their actions are unselfish. Piliavin and Charng argue that "the data from sociology, economics, political science, and social psychology are all at least compatible with the position that altruism is part of human nature."[20] This line of research is united by its identification of altruism as a robust form of action that can become rooted in individuals' basic motivations and identities. The details of the explanations for altruism vary somewhat, ranging from arguments for a universal trait of empathy to theories of the emergence of altruistic identity over time.[21]

In keeping with these broad trends, most research on organ donation and procurement has focused on questions of individual motivation and costs. It tries to discover the sources of opposition to donation and ways of overcoming them. Most research on organ shortage finds that refusals happen because of bad information or myths about the donation process; in other words, irrational beliefs and fears about organ donation may be responsible for keeping the procurement rate down.[22] "The shortage of donated organs is not due to lack of knowledge or awareness of the plight of would-be recipients. Instead, the problem arises from factors such as unstated motivations, perceived risks, and unarticulated fears about donation."[23] For those working with a concept of altruism as motivated action, the issue is treated as an problem at the level of the individual, the solution to which lies in understanding (and perhaps adjusting) the motives of potential donors. For those who are skeptical of motivational altruism but nevertheless retain an individual-level point of view, the solution is to change the payoffs to donors—most likely, by financially reimbursing them.

The context created by organizations and institutions tends to be absent from this approach, whether the topic is altruism in general or organ donation in particular. Much of the experimental work on motivated altruism examines how people react to the unexpected chance to immediately help a stranger who is clearly in need of assistance.[24] Studies of help "in the context of a relationship are largely absent in this tradition."[25] Although research has solidly established that "the altruistic impulse does exist,"[26] it has less to say about how this impulse is institutionalized and managed. Neither does it explore the possibility that altruistic acts that are rare from an individual's point of view might be routine from an organization's perspective.

Altruistic action often happens in response to a direct request. Studies of charitable giving emphasize that "communities of participation" and direct requests are necessary to channel personal values, prior dispositions, and available resources into actual donations.[27] Organizations may formalize this process. Peter Frumkin notes that "while volunteers remain an important engine driving nonprofits, most nonprofits use professionals to manage volunteers, rather than using volunteers to manage their organizations."[28] Studies of the nonprofit and voluntary sector have shown that organizations respond to changes in their environment, both by conforming to externally imposed regulations and strategically working to change that environment.[29] If such organizations are actively engaged in soliciting altruism, these strategies may affect how well this task is accomplished.

As with research on motivated altruism in general, researchers have discovered (and rediscovered) the importance of situational factors to organ donation without systematically pursuing them. An important early study by Roberta Simmons found that living kidney donors were more likely to have been asked in person to give than were nondonors.[30] A more recent study found that female relatives were more likely to donate a kidney than were male relatives, possibly because women were more likely than men to be asked to donate.[31] In the case of cadaveric donors, the importance of the person-to-person request process has been subject to increasing attention from researchers.[32]

We can think of variation in rates of organ procurement, then, as being shaped by two kinds of forces: features of OPOs' catchment areas and characteristics of the OPOs themselves. The research literature on organ donation and donor motivation suggests that even when we control for causes of death, facts about social structure and demography will still affect the procurement rate.[33] In particular, population density, racial composition, the poverty rate, and the average degree of educational attainment in an OPO region might all be important.

POPULATION DENSITY. Some OPOs administer relatively small, densely populated regions. Others service huge areas. While the New York Organ Donor Network procures donors from the millions of people concentrated in the five boroughs of New York City, the territory of the LifeCenter Northwest Donor Network includes nearly all of Washington, Idaho, Montana, and Alaska. Potential donors must be located quickly and transported to a suitable hospital. This is easier to accomplish in a densely populated area. If OPOs are responsible for large, sparsely populated regions, their procurement efforts may well be focused on any more densely populated areas within it. Even so, the number of donors procured per thousand evaluable deaths will most likely be lower.

RACE. Support for organ donation varies a great deal by race. Blacks are less likely to donate than whites, less likely to sign donor cards or discuss donation with their families, and less likely to support the idea of organ donation generally.[34] At the individual level, African American families refuse consent to procure organs at much higher rates than members of other ethnic groups, and there is evidence that their refusals are rooted in a set of concerns that differ from those of white families.[35] Beliefs that the transplant system is unfair to minorities, a more general distrust of the medical system, or ineffective methods of request on the part of OPOs have all been suggested as possible explanations.[36] The general position of African Americans in the transplant system is also relevant. Recent studies have found that blacks face several structural barriers to organ transplantation. Incidence of hypertension and end-stage renal disease is highest in the black population, and African Americans comprise 34 percent of those on dialysis and 30 percent of those waiting for kidney transplants.[37] Yet blacks are much less likely than whites to express an interest in, be listed for, or receive a transplant.[38] As it stands, the reluctance to donate among minorities is a fact of OPOs' operating environments. The higher the percentage of African Americans in an OPO's service population, the lower its procurement rate is likely to be.

POVERTY RATE. When a potential donor becomes available, procurement must happen quickly. If the donor is an accident victim, she must be found and brought to a hospital quickly and placed on a ventilator. A procurement team must be able to get to the hospital quickly and do the surgery to procure the organs. The better the facility the more efficient the process will be. OPOs that serve wealthier areas are more likely to have the right resources and facilities available to them and the hospitals they work with. We should therefore expect that OPOs serving poorer counties will tend to procure fewer of the potential donors that become available.

EDUCATION. Survey data show a higher level of support for organ donation among more educated people.[39] As discussed above, there is a gap between abstract support for organ donation and the actual decision as a next of kin to allow procurement to go ahead. But on the whole its effect should be positive: we should still expect OPOs serving more educated populations to do better on average than others, because they ought to encounter fewer obstacles when attempting to secure consent from donor families.

Despite their importance, these structural and demographic forces cannot be the whole story. Of central interest to us is the role played by the OPOs themselves. We can think of three broad features of an organization that will affect its ability to accomplish its goals. These are its resources or overall budget; its scope or reach within its environment; and its policies and practices as it carries out its task.

ORGANIZATIONAL RESOURCES. Were there no OPOs, there would be no organ donors. Donor procurement is a resource-intensive procedure requiring rapid and coordinated organizational action. Dedicated facilities for procurement make the process more efficient on a number of measures.[40] The point should generalize. Larger, resource-rich OPOs should be expected to do better on average than smaller ones. We can use OPO administrative spending per annum to capture this idea. When measured relative to the number of potential donors, OPO spending indexes the resources that the organization brings to the procurement process.

ORGANIZATIONAL SCOPE. OPOs are not the only players in the procurement process. Most donor-evaluable deaths occur in hospitals. In some cases, the OPO will have a staff member working at the hospital. More often, a member of the hospital staff has the task of contacting the OPO to let them know that a potential donor has become available. Hospitals thus play a key role in the procurement process.[41] OPOs may make referral agreements with hospitals. The more hospitals an OPO has referral agreements with, the more donors it is likely to procure. This is a measure of an OPO's reach, or scope. Separate from spending, it captures the extent of the OPO's coverage and the range of its ties to potential sites of donor procurement. Because not all hospitals will have the right kind of patients, we count the number of referrers per thousand in-hospital evaluable deaths.

ORGANIZATIONAL POLICY. Beyond their varied resources and reach, OPOs differ in their procurement policies and consent practices. Although all OPOs are interested in getting people to carry donor cards, donor families are central to the procurement process, as it is they who give or refuse consent for donation.[42] Convincing families to agree to donation is a delicate affair.[43] Successful organ procurement should be related to the strategies adopted by OPOs. This idea is consistent with broader social-science research that seeks to situate altruism within an organizational and institutional framework and with other findings about charitable donation, which have shown that whether and how one is asked to give is a better predictor of giving than the individual characteristics of donors.[44] Within the transplant field, researchers find that families rarely suggest donation of their own accord and that "educational interventions for health care professionals and a coordinated requesting process that includes the organ procurement organization and hospital personnel result in a higher number of donations."[45]

OPOs differ in their policies regarding whether and how families or next of kin are asked for permission to donate. Although in principle (and in law) a signed organ donor card is sufficient to justify procurement, in practice, as we have noted, the situation is more fluid. There is substantial variation in consent policies.[46] Specifically, OPOs vary in how willing they say they are to try to obtain consent. Some, for example, may be more willing than others to suggest that the wishes of the deceased be respected even if the family has reservations about donating. The expectation is that the stronger the policy, the higher the procurement rate.[47]

The results of a regression model of the main environmental and organizational predictors of procurement are shown in figure 3.5. (A more detailed summary can be found in table A.1 in the appendix.) The vertical lines show the predicted effect of moving a variable from its 25th percentile to its 75th percentile. The shaded horizontal bars show a range of confidence intervals for each prediction, with the very ends of the bars measuring a 99 percent interval. So, for example, the effect on an OPO of increasing the size of the black population from 2.67 percent to 11.4 percent is to lower the percentage of donors procured per thousand evaluable deaths by about three points. Increasing the percentage of poor people from 12.5 to 18.9 percent lowers the procurement rate by almost four points. These negative effects are consistent with our expectations.

Also as expected, increasing the population density has a strongly pos-

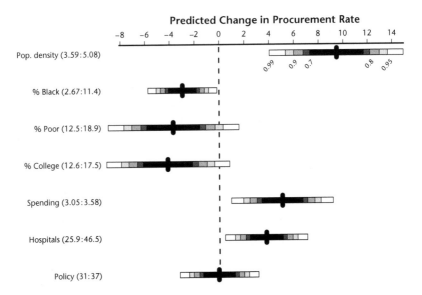

Figure 3.5. Effects of environmental and organizational variables on procurement rates
Notes: For each variable, the vertical line represents the predicted percentage change in the procurement rate if the variable changes from its 25th percentile to its 75th percentile value. (The actual 25th and 75th percentile values are shown to the right of each variable's label.) The shaded ranges around the predicted values mark confidence intervals ranging from 70 to 99 percent.

itive effect on procurement. People are very unevenly distributed across OPOs, so the model represented in figure 3.5 uses the logarithm of the population density, which smooths out the distribution. This makes the predicted effect look somewhat bigger than it really is, as moving from the 25th to the 75th percentile of a log distribution represents a large percentage change in the underlying variable. A 10 percent increase in population per square mile increases the procurement rate by just over 0.6 of a point.

Increasing the percentage of the population that is college educated has a negative effect on procurement. This is unexpected, as we know that there is substantially stronger support than average for organ donation among more educated people. Nevertheless, it is not clear that this effect would show up here, given that we are measuring effects at the OPO rather than the individual level. We might think that better-educated people are less likely to die in circumstances conducive to procurement—in automobile accidents, for example, or from gunshot or stab wounds. Recall, however, that the outcome measure is the procurement rate among evaluable deaths, rather than all deaths or the live population. Selection into the donor pool is therefore already controlled for and cannot explain the negative effect of education.[48] One possibility is that the effect is the result of outlying observations. Education is more sensitive than the other variables to the presence of a small number of cases in the data, but even when these cases are dropped one by one its effect remains negative. The finding seems robust given the data but remains to be fully explained.

Taken together, the environmental variables explain about a third of the observed variation in the procurement rate. When we add in the three organizational measures, we can explain more than half of the variance. These measures show some interesting effects. OPO spending per capita is positively and significantly related to the procurement rate. (As with population density, we use the logarithm of spending here.) A 10 percent increase in spending raises the procurement rate by nearly nine-tenths of a point. The number of referring hospitals per thousand evaluable deaths also has a strong effect on procurement. A 5 percentage point increase in the density of referrers raises the procurement rate by about a three-quarters of a point. These results strongly suggest that the organizational resources of OPOs play a very important role in determining the procurement rate.

In contrast, the measure of OPO policy shows no strong effects. The variable measures an OPO's willingness to procure in hypothetical circumstances where consent is ambiguous. The consent policies of OPOs have been assumed to play an important role in the procurement process, so it is surprising to see so little effect here. Two interpretations suggest themselves. It may be that in fact the consent policies of OPOs do not have a strong effect on the procurement rate. The original survey instrument took considerable care to ensure accurate responses, however. A second interpretation is that, although the survey is accurate as far as it goes, it did not pick out real organizational practices. Discussion of hard cases, whether hypothetical or real, is a staple of the bioethics literature, and of course teasing out these cases can teach us about the scope and limits of our ethical ideas. But these kind of dilemmas may have little to do with the everyday work of organ procurement. What-if questions about the limits of procurement policy might not be a helpful way to understand what is happening inside OPOs.

Evidence from other sources supports this idea. From the mid-1980s to the mid-1990s, the South Carolina Organ Procurement Agency (SCOPA) consistently ranked in the bottom half of OPOs in terms of procurement rates. This was partly due to its geographical location, a poorer than average area with a higher than average black population. Our findings so far in this chapter make its poor performance unsurprising. Since 1997, however, this OPO has increased its donation rate by 83 percent as a result of a series of changes in the management of the procurement process.[49] Consistent with the ideas developed in this chapter, SCOPA invested more money and people in the procurement process, increasing its field staff from eight to twenty-one employees. But it also changed its procurement methods. The key innovation was to decouple the moment donor families were told about the brain death of the patient from the moment they were asked to consent to donation. Tasks previously assigned to a single procurement coordinator—hospital liason, family support counselor, donor clinician, recovery coordinator, and aftercare coordinator—were assigned to separate employees, each with an appropriate professional background. The OPO's organizational mission had been simply to procure as many high-quality donor organs as possible. During the restructuring, SCOPA changed its name to LifePoint and added a "family support service." The goal of this part of the organization was "to insure that families of dying patients . . . made well-informed decisions about donation and had timely bereavement counseling and follow-up."[50] A crucial aspect of the reorganization was that the person who explained to families that their loved one was brain dead, and who spent a considerable amount of time (perhaps a whole day) helping them with this realization, was no longer the person who requested consent for donation. Within five years of the new methods' introduction, consent rates were about 85 percent, close to the proportion of the population that survey data suggests supports organ donation in the first place.

The implications of these organizational changes are striking. On the narrow question of the measurement of OPO policy, they suggest that asking detailed questions about an OPO's willingness to procure donors under adverse circumstances (e.g., in the face of opposition from the families) might not be very informative. LifePoint's success was due to strategies designed to make it easier for shocked and grieving families to understand and fully support the procurement process. By splitting the information-provider role from the consent-request role, they ensured that the person providing families with information about brain death (and helping them manage for the day in the hospital) would not be perceived as having an ulterior motive. Thus, families are carefully managed by the organization in a way that shepherds them toward the vital moment when consent is requested.

These results show the value of looking at organ donation as an organizational problem. Donation is an exceptional, one-shot event for donor families, but it is a stable and mostly predictable circumstance from an organizational point of view. It depends on exogenous environmental forces, but it is also strongly affected by the resources and scope of the procurement agency. The social production of altruistic action—the provision of a stable supply of voluntarily donated hearts, livers, and other organs—can be thought of as a resource-extraction problem that organizations solve more or less effectively. From this perspective, the individual capacity for altruism and the social organization of procurement are not separate questions but rather two aspects of the same process. As organizations create "contexts for giving" they elicit altruistic action differentially across populations. Rather than simply discovering preexisting populations with dispositions to give, they help create their own donor pool.

Understanding how organizations acquire donors is essential to understanding how exercising one's capacity for altruism becomes a routine event in a stable system of exchange. We find a similar idea in recent studies of voluntary association and civic participation, which develop the view that "involvement in volunteer activities does not simply spring from already constituted social groups or from aggregated individual characteristics" but is structured by institutions.[51] A onetime event like organ donation would seem to be the most likely case where this argument would *not* apply, where either the distinctive characteristics of individual altruists or the motivating force of generalized norms would be most important. But this need be true only if one-shot exchanges must, by definition, lack an institutional context. The presence of chronically repeated actions or widespread routine is usually a good measure of institutionalization. Rare events seem less susceptible to institutional control by their very nature. But we need to look for routines in the right place. For events like organ donation, we must separate the frequency of individual altruistic action from the degree to which the *context* for that action is socially organized. This allows us to see how rare or even once-off events may nevertheless be managed in a well-organized social environment. In this way, we can gain leverage on the question of why rates of different kinds of altruistic action vary.

————

In chapter 2, I argued that transplant advocates in the United States have successfully made organ procurement seem normal and morally worthwhile. Normal, because they helped turn a difficult and potentially controversial process into something you can assent to in principle on the back of your driver's license. Morally worthwhile, because they encouraged a public account of donation centered on heroic individuals (both donors and recipients) and generous families giving the gift of life to those in need. In this chapter, we have moved away from the public and cultural work of account building and focused on the logistical effort that OPOs put into the procurement process. The aim is to show how organ procurement functions as a large exchange system, and to move toward explaining variation in procurement rates within the system from a structural and organizational perspective.

Kidneys move between OPOs and hospitals in predominantly regional exchange networks centered on major transplant centers. Big importers are often located next to big exporters. Larger, more sparsely populated areas tend to have an even balance of trade or may export a small number of organs to regions with larger transplant programs. A few regions manage to procure a large number of organs and export many of them, even when they have their own busy transplant centers.

Procurement rates also display strong regional patterns, with the upper Midwest in particular supplying far more donors than average, with most of the West and South doing poorly by comparison. Some of this variation has to do with the ecological features of OPO service areas—their population density, proportion of African Americans, poverty rates, and so on. But the analysis also showed that the resources and scope of the organizations themselves play a very important role in determining how many organs are procured. Two of the three organizational measures showed strong effects: Investment in the logistics of procurement (as measured by administrative spending and the number of connections to hospitals) has a significant influence on the number of organs procured.

Given the available data, it is difficult to parse the precise relationship between individual and environmental effects in a definitive way. Individual motives and preferences may lurk behind environmental measures. The education, poverty, and race variables might represent population-based measures of individual-level preferences, for example. The results for measures of race (in particular) and poverty are consistent with individual-level explanations for their effects. The education effect goes against received wisdom on support for donation. This could mean we need to reassess our views about the relationship between preferences and decisions at the individual level rather than introduce a new structural explanation. Alternatively, the causal mechanisms might be working at the organizational level, as education levels are tied to the way potential donors become available.

Neither the standard cultural account of donation nor most existing research have much to say beyond the question of individual motives and the immediate moment of request. Yet taken together, structural and organizational characteristics of the procurement system explain half of the observed variation in collection rates. Putting altruism in its institutional context does not amount to begging the question of where it comes from in the first place, however. We can agree that if people simply had no inclination to be altruistic, then it would never be observed. Similarly, if altruism was not a sustainable way of acting, it would only ever be a rare or sporadic event. But many empirically interesting forms of altruism are widespread, stable, and well institutionalized. Insofar as we want to explain what we observe, altruism cannot be properly understood without reference to this context. Confining ourselves to individual motives will not do.

There is no need to create a false opposition between individual actions and organizational practices. Individual donors and their families have reasons to give. But procurement organizations provide the context in which the next of kin can be asked about donation. In the longer term, they help create a body of publicly available reasons that makes giving consent sensible and appropriate. Without the logistical effort that makes it possible to donate, possessing the necessary willingness to give would not have any practical consequences. Without the reasons that make it meaningful to give, providing the necessary opportunities to donate would be futile. As a plausible cultural account of donation is established, and as OPOs efficiently acquire potential donors, more and more people find themselves with the motive to give, the means to account for it, and the opportunity to do it.

FOUR

Collection Regimes and Donor Populations

Organ donation usually happens when the next of kin of an accident victim agrees to a medical team's request. As we have seen, it is a difficult business that requires enormous sensitivity and effort. Like organs, blood is scarce and valuable, and yet is supplied by voluntary donors who receive nothing for their trouble. It carries much of the same cultural significance as a gift of one's own body, but is something most people could do with just a little effort, if they wanted to. It has therefore been seen as "perhaps the purest example" of altruistic behavior.[1] Its symbolic resonance—an anonymous gift of life to an unknown recipient—only makes it more likely to be mentioned in the same breath as altruism or volunteering.[2] Those in charge of the blood supply routinely stress that very few people give blood, and so we tend to think of donors as special people. The surprisingly small research literature on blood donation generally shares this view and as with organ donation asks what makes donors special.[3] For all these reasons, blood donors provide the perfect example to those interested in attacking the self-interested utility maximizer of neoclassical economics. *Homo economicus* wouldn't give blood unless he was paid enough money; real-life donors do not reason in this way.

This chapter continues the argument that I have been developing in the previous two chapters, broadening its scope from organizational variation within a single country to cross-national institutional differences. The central idea remains the same. As economic sociologists have been arguing since the 1980s, patterns in the organization of exchange must be understood by examining the social-structural framework that provides the incentives, opportunities, and constraints that actors think and work with. Although this point should apply equally well both to altruistic and selfish action, the moral and rhetorical attractions of blood donation have insulated it from scrutiny. The institutional underpinnings of the blood supply have been almost entirely overshadowed by the image of the individual altruist. In contrast, I argue that as with organs, blood can be seen not so much as something that individuals donate but as something that organizations collect.

All industrialized countries have a strong and permanent demand for blood. Large parts of their medical systems would quickly collapse without it. Everything from emergency paramedical care to routine operations would become difficult or impossible. In addition, many people's lives depend on a constant supply of blood products. But different countries choose to meet this demand in different ways. Some manage to collect much more blood per capita than others, and they get it from different kinds of people. Some countries have a relatively small pool of regular donors, others a larger group of occasional suppliers. If the blood supply simply relied on the goodwill of individual altruists, it is not clear why such variation should exist. Yet there has been next to no empirical investigation of these cross-national differences.

In this chapter I analyze a large survey that contains information on patterns of blood donation in the European Union. I describe and discuss blood collection practices within the E.U. and identify three relevant sources of variation, in order of importance. First, the organization in charge of collecting blood in each country. There are three main kinds, namely the state, the Red Cross, and independent blood banks. Second, whether a volunteer donor group exists within a country. And third, the presence or absence of for-profit plasma collection. The analysis shows that there are stable patterns of variation across different systems: different organizations collect their blood from different kinds of people. Moreover, the act of blood donation looks quite different under different systems. For example, Red Cross regimes seem to collect more blood from young, unmarried people than do systems run by independent blood banks or the state.

The Elusive Altruist

The need for a comparative, institutional perspective on blood donation can be seen from the findings of the existing literature on individual donors. Studies generally try to establish the demographic characteristics and motivations of donors. When asked, most donors will offer some altruistic reason for giving, often citing feelings of community attachment or commitment to the common good as their motive. Researchers have tried to correlate these motives with the demographic characteristics of the donors.[4] We know there are some strictly individual constraints on donation. Women give blood less often than men for medical reasons. Women are lighter than men on average and are also more prone to anemia (and pregnancy). Each of these conditions disqualifies one from donating, so there are fewer women in the pool of potential donors. Older people are also more likely to be excluded from the donor pool for medical reasons. This does not explain why the better-off and better-educated give more. Nor does it explain why relatively few eligible people give in the first place. The motives of donors are clearly important but should not stop us from asking how the institutional setting—the organization of recruitment, collection, and publicity—might make it more or less difficult for some kinds of people to donate blood.

Studies of donor motivation do sometimes recognize the role of institutions, though their research design usually prevents them from investigating them properly. Asking how more blood might be collected, some research has recommended changing the structure of incentives offered to donors, as opposed to searching ever harder for the elusive altruists.[5] Jane Piliavin and Peter Callero followed first-time donors over time and developed an analysis of how a person grows into a "donor-role."[6] But they also recognize that other, nonindividual factors are important. They provide evidence that both personal networks and simple organizational differences have important effects on donation rates. If many of your friends are donors, you are likely to be a donor as well. The accessibility of blood centers—whether collection points are mobile or fixed, for example—also affects whether people give. However, their research design confines them to the United States, and so the effect of large-scale institutional variation is outside the scope of their study.

The findings from this literature are easy to summarize. Studies have found a reliable "modal profile" for blood donors and a similarly typical pattern of altruistic motives.[7] On the basis of these studies, the expected demographic characteristics of individual donors can be summed up by saying that the typical donor is a male in his early thirties, and that the odds of donating blood increase with educational attainment and income.

Research also suggests that people are more likely to donate blood if they know other donors or if they know people who have received transfusions (or other blood products). Similarly, a study by Alvin Drake and his collaborators found that those who are "close to blood needs" were more likely to donate.[8] We should therefore expect a network effect: if all your friends are blood donors, you are likely to be one too. If you know a hemophiliac, you should also be more likely to have given blood at some point.

Blood Collection Regimes

Individual motives for giving blood must be set in the context of institutionalized methods for collecting it. Richard Titmuss's *The Gift Relationship* remains the most influential study of cross-national institutional variation in the blood supply and is almost the only example of its kind.[9] I discuss some of the difficulties with Titmuss's arguments about the relative quality of blood in volunteer and for-profit systems in the next chapter. His emphasis on the consequences of variation in the social organization of the blood supply, however, was fundamentally correct. For Titmuss, it was the structure of the health system, not the psychology of donors, that was crucial to the composition of the donor pool.

In spite of a common European Union policy encouraging voluntary blood donation, we find that rates of donation and modes of organization differ considerably across countries. Figure 4.1 shows the percentage of people in thirteen countries who have ever given blood, as reported in the 1993 Eurobarometer survey.[10] The rates range from 14 percent in Luxembourg to 44 percent next door in France. This wide variation in donation rates is interesting. Why should there be 20 or 30 percentage points difference between France and Greece, on the one hand, and Luxembourg and Portugal, on the other? If we think of donation as purely a question of individual motivation, it seems unlikely that the individual propensity to generosity should change quite so abruptly at national borders. We should also be wary of writing the difference off to cultural variation, particularly given that countries that we might expect to fall together culturally (France and Luxembourg, Denmark and Norway) have dissimilar donation rates.

Individual-level explanations cannot properly account for this variation. We should look beyond the psychology of giving to the social organization of the blood supply. As noted above, there are three relevant

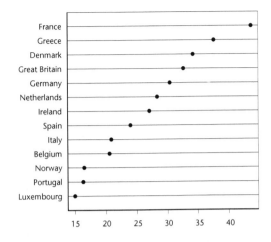

Figure 4.1. Percent of the population who have ever given blood, by country

institutional features of the blood supply that vary across Europe: the collection regime, the presence of volunteer donor organizations, and the presence of for-profit plasma collection.

A directive issued in 1989 committed the European Union to securing its supply of whole blood and plasma from voluntary, unpaid donors. This mandate, however, said nothing about the kind of organization that should do the collecting. At the same time, the Council of Europe commissioned a series of research papers on blood suppliers that were later published as white papers.[11] One of these is based on interviews with those responsible for the blood and plasma supply in each E.U. member state and describes the different sorts of organization that exist within these countries.

Broadly speaking, there are three types of blood collection regime in Europe:[12]

1. In the United Kingdom, France, and Ireland a National Health Service or state-run blood organization has a monopoly on blood collection. These countries have no other collection agencies.

2. The Red Cross has a monopoly in Belgium, Luxembourg, and the Netherlands and controls the majority of collection in Germany (with a minority held by hospital or community blood banks).

3. Blood banks control a majority of collection (with a minority held by the Red Cross) in Greece, Italy, Norway, Portugal, and Spain. Denmark is the only country where banks have a monopoly.

While precise data on market shares would have been ideal, information was available only about the relative predominance of the Red Cross and blood banks in those countries where they share responsibility for the supply.[13]

Volunteer donor organizations are a second important distinguishing feature. Donors are organized into one or more national associations in Denmark, France, Greece, Italy. and Spain. Denmark's organization, for example, "was founded in 1932 when a boy-scout movement established a corps of young adult boy-scouts who on a voluntary non-remunerated basis were willing to be called to hospitals to donate blood."[14] The Voluntary Blood Donors of Denmark supply hospitals with donors. In return, hospitals pay the local organization a small fee per donation, which is used for publicity and further recruitment efforts.

Italy has a slightly different form of organization. Instead of sending donors to hospitals the organizations collect the blood themselves and send it to hospitals. In this they resemble community blood banks. The majority of blood banks in Italy are run by one of three donor organizations, which are organized in different parts of the country and do not compete with one another. The largest claims about eight hundred thousand members.[15]

France, which has a state-run system, and Spain, where collection is organized by blood banks, also have important donor organizations. In my analysis, therefore, we may distinguish between a blood-banking system and the presence of a voluntary donor group, even though in some countries the donor groups may have a hand in running the blood banks.

For-profit plasma collection is the third feature. Much of the debate about blood has contrasted the dangers of commercialism with the virtues of voluntarism. While all blood suppliers sell blood products to hospitals or to one another, Europe has essentially no individual market for blood of the kind that existed in the United States in the 1960s. The commercial collection and processing of plasma is the main exception to this rule. Plasma can be extracted from whole blood or obtained separately through plasmapheresis. Plasmapheresis takes longer than donating a unit of blood. It can also be done much more often: the body replaces lost plasma much faster than it does lost blood.

Plasma and whole blood collection overlap in complicated ways. In general, although nonprofit blood suppliers may collect plasma from voluntary donors, they do not process it any further. It is either used directly (as with whole blood) or sold to commercial plasma fractionators. Practices vary. Denmark, for example, has a state-run fractionation plant (although its capacity is small compared to the country's other, commercial plant). The only exceptions of interest here are those countries where a company buys plasma directly from individual suppliers (rather than in bulk from regular blood suppliers who obtain it from donors). Spain and Germany each have such a system. The world market for plasma is dominated by the United States. A number of U.S. companies buy plasma from individuals, serving both domestic and export markets. But in Europe, the commercial market for plasma suppliers is quite small and concentrated. People are much less likely to be plasma donors, or especially plasma sellers, than blood donors.

With this information about the structure of the European Union's blood supply, we are in a position to work out some ideas about the way in which characteristics of collection organizations in each country might affect the number and characteristics of blood donors. We can think of blood donation as a special kind of volunteering that involves more than just money or time.[16] Indeed, the physical and symbolic nature of the gift of blood is what makes it attractive as the perfect example of altruistic giving. How similar blood donation really is to regular volunteering is partly an empirical question (which I examine below), but it is close enough to suggest that what we know about other kinds of volunteering might also apply to blood.

One possibility is that the link is quite direct, that a country's blood donation rate will line up with its rate of volunteering. We might expect countries with generally high rates of voluntary activity to also have high rates of blood donation. Andrew Greeley discusses the best available data for Europe, which come from the 1991 wave of the European Values Survey.[17] He notes that "church attendance and membership in religious organizations correlate with volunteering [in Europe]. . . . Even in countries where religious activity is not high, as in the Scandinavian countries, religious behavior still has a significant impact on voluntary service."[18] His data, together with other research, suggest that involvement in organized religious activity encourages both religious and secular forms of volunteering.[19] The same might be true for blood donation.

This correlation between participation in religious activity and other forms of volunteering takes us a step closer to answering the question of the role of organizations. In general, blood is collected by public or nonprofit organizations that solicit voluntary donations from individuals. Why might some forms of organization be better than others at doing this? Research on how organizations solicit money shows that rates of giving tend to increase with age. Educational attainment also usually has a positive effect.[20] But the most consistent finding in this literature is organizational rather than individual: being asked to contribute is one of the most important determinants of giving in general.[21] And although there are better and worse ways to ask, simply giving someone the opportunity to volunteer can be decisive. The staff of nonprofit and voluntary organizations are often well aware of the importance of "the Ask"—the moment when a gift or donation is solicited. A survey of American blood donors carried out in 1975 confirms this general finding. As in other studies, when asked why they gave blood, donors tended to give altruistic reasons. But when nondonors were asked why they had never donated, the two most common responses were "I was never asked" and "There was no convenient opportunity." Poor organization—rather than selfish motivation—kept people from giving.[22]

We should expect some collection regimes to do better than others, depending on the opportunities for giving that they offer. This suggests the potential importance of other social or organizational contexts that might make it easier to tap potential donors. Someone who is currently a student, for instance, is more likely to be recruited in a campus blood drive. Union membership might have similar effects if blood collection is organized through workplace drives. General demographic characteristics like age and educational attainment should change the likelihood of being a blood donor in ways already seen in previous research, but situational or contextual variables that pick out a recruitment mechanism ought to matter as well.

Larger, better funded organizations will be in a position to publicize their needs more broadly than smaller, more disaggregated ones. The publicity efforts of large organizations also benefit from economies of scale, from name recognition, and from the trust they engender. (The Red Cross symbol is instantly recognized the world over.) Large organizations may also find it easier to coordinate effective recruitment drives and can invest their time in areas where they know the number of donors is large. For these reasons, in our case, we should expect the Red Cross to be better than blood banks at attracting donors.

If simply reaching potential donors is what matters, then countries where the state has a monopoly on collection might do best of all. Other things being equal, a national system is likely to be better funded, have a wider coverage, and have more recruitment options open to it than other kinds of organization. Operating within a national health system, the blood-collection organization should find it easier to integrate its activities into the general package of benefits provided by the state. Giving blood might more easily be seen—as Titmuss argued—as part of a general quid pro quo, part of the individual obligation incurred by receipt of the public goods provided by the state. State systems should also have an easier time getting access to other state organizations where donors might be found (such as universities and the civil service). The resources to run large-scale recruitment efforts may also be more readily available to state-run collection agencies.

Blood-banking systems are by nature more disaggregated than either state-run or Red Cross systems. The collection regime is made up of a number of blood banks, often tied to local hospitals, usually self-administered, and always serving some local population. This does not imply that blood banks will do worse than larger alternatives, although they should show more variation. Some local banks will be better run than others. In addition, blood banks offer a wider range of incentives to donors than either Red Cross or state systems. Some use an insurance system, in which donors build up credit for their own operations by donating regularly themselves. Banking systems are also more likely to offer autologous donations, allowing patients to build up a stock of their own blood solely for personal use. This variability in organizational style and incentive systems should be reflected in collection rates.

What about the pernicious effects of commercialism? Titmuss argued that paid suppliers would drive out volunteers. Given that the blood supply today is essentially voluntary, it is difficult to test this claim, especially for European countries. The best we can do is to examine whether countries with a commercial plasma sector differ from those without one. Because whole blood collection is almost never commercialized, though the plasma supply may be, the opportunity to donate voluntarily always exists. By Titmuss's logic, we should nonetheless expect at least some variation tied to income from plasma sales. But because the plasma sector is not a major force in the European blood collection system, we should not be surprised if its effect is difficult to pin down.

Conversely, five countries in the sample have volunteer donor organizations that are committed to the ideal of altruism. We saw that one of the main findings in studies of individual donors is that, while there is a "modal donor," many who fit this profile do not donate. I suggest that donor organizations will find it easiest to recruit from this particular group of nondonors. Thus, if the modal donor is a well-educated male, a donor group will find it easiest to recruit from among the many well-educated males who would not otherwise donate. This will skew the donor population toward the modal profile rather than increasing the odds of donation by atypical individuals. Where a donor organization exists, people already likely to donate blood should be even more likely to do so, but those now unlikely to donate will be less likely to do so.

The discussion so far has identified some individual characteristics and institutional features that ought to make blood donation more likely. We have also seen how donation rates vary widely across countries, together with some preliminary evidence that this variation is systematic and that collection regimes might play a role in the structure of a country's donor population. To get a better sense of the structure of blood donation in these countries, we can construct some models of the donation rate using the Eurobarometer survey data.

Variation across Countries

To begin with, we can look just at the role of individual-level characteristics in predicting blood donation in different countries.[23] Our existing knowledge about the makeup of donor populations is broadly confirmed, but the basic pattern varies substantially across countries. For example, on average women are about half as likely as men to have donated, but although a significant gap is found in every country its size varies substantially. It is narrowest in Norway, Britain, and Ireland. In these countries, women are about 70 percent as likely to have given as men. In Greece, Portugal, and Italy, by contrast, women are only about 15 to 30 percent as likely as men to have donated.

We also expected that the odds of donating would increase with ties to transfusion recipients, educational attainment, and income. Network ties to blood recipients have a strongly positive effect in seven countries, raising the odds of having donated by, on average, about a third. The effect is strongest in Germany, where an additional tie makes donation 1.7 times more likely. This is probably a result of a collection system that strongly encourages or obliges people who have operations scheduled to have their relatives give blood. Network effects are weak or absent in Britain, Ireland, Italy, Spain, Denmark, and Luxembourg. Britain shows by far the weakest effect of network ties. The effect of education on donation is largest in Ireland and France, where each additional year of education raises the odds of having given by about 12 percent. We also see significant though smaller effects in Germany, Belgium, Denmark, and Norway, with about a 3 to 4 percent increase in the odds of donation. The Mediterranean countries and Portugal show no significant education effects. Lastly, moving up a notch in the income distribution significantly raises the odds of donation, by about 6 percent on average, with the strongest effects seen in Norway (almost 20 percent) and Ireland (16 percent). There are no significant income effects in Britain, the Netherlands, Belgium, Spain, and Italy.

In addition to the size of the total donor population we are interested in those people who have given blood in the past year. Regular donors form a much smaller group than those who have given at some stage in their lives. Now, in principle it might be the case that the personal characteristics that predict ever having given blood also predict whether someone is a recent donor. But it is more likely that additional mechanisms are also at work. It turns out that if we try to predict recent donation using the variables that we have been discussing, both the effects and their interpretation change, and some new variables become more important. We have seen that in every country being female significantly lowers the odds of ever having given blood, by about half on average. But in several countries this gender gap disappears when we look only at recent donors. Britain, France, Belgium, the Netherlands, Denmark, Norway, and Spain show no significant difference among those who have given in the past year.[24] Similarly, education and income do not predict recent donation across countries as well as they predict ever having given blood. This is consistent with the idea that general sociodemographic characteristics do not pick out regular donors as well as measures situated in some organizational context. For instance, being a member of a union significantly raises the odds of recent donation in Scandinavia, Belgium, France, Germany, and Italy but is not strongly associated with ever having given. Similarly, regular church attendance is sigificantly associated with having given blood in the past year but does not predict whether a person has ever given blood.

We also expected that countries with high rates of volunteering would also have high rates of blood donation. To test this idea, I compared national volunteering rates calculated from the 1991 European Values Survey (EVS) to blood donation rates calculated from the data analyzed in this chapter.[25] Across all countries, there is no correlation between the volunteering rate and the proportion of the population who had given blood in the previous year.[26] In Red Cross countries, however, the general volunteering rate (measured by the EVS) and the blood donation rate are strongly correlated, though as we saw above that there is no association between them in general.[27]

Blood Collection in Institutional Context

As rates of blood donation vary across countries, so does the nature of the relationship between donation and individual characteristics like gender or education. Might this cross-national variation be systematically related to the social organization of the blood supply? Figure 4.2 shows three mea-

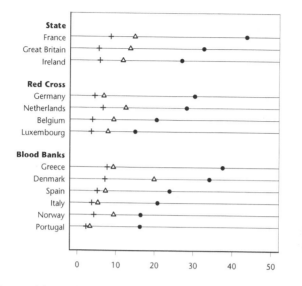

Figure 4.2. Percent of the population who have given blood in the last year (+), who have given many times (▲), and who have ever given (●), ordered by regime type.

sures of the donor pool, arranged by collection regime. The broadest is the percentage of people in each country who say they have ever given blood. State-run regimes tend toward the upper end of the overall range, with Red Cross countries scoring below them. Blood-banking regimes show the widest variation. If we look at those who say they have donated many times in the past (as opposed to never, once, or just a few times), state regimes again seem to do slightly better than Red Cross countries, on the whole. Denmark has the highest percentage of regular donors and stands out from the other blood-banking regimes in this respect. (The ratio between regular donors and those who have ever given is highest in Denmark, followed by Norway.) Patterns are harder to discern among those who have given in the past year, because the numbers are smaller, though again Red Cross countries may do a little worse than state-run systems, with blood-banking regimes displaying the widest range. Interestingly, the southern European blood-banking countries (Italy, Greece, Spain, and Portugal) show the smallest gap between recent and regular givers—in these countries, recent donors are more likely to say they are also regular donors.

We can estimate the institutional effects and their effect on individual characteristics in a more formal way, while controlling for variation at the national level. We keep the individual-level variables as before and add measures of the social organization of blood donation in each country, namely the collection regime and the presence or absence of donor groups.[28] The main finding is that donation patterns in state-run, Red Cross, and blood-banking regimes differ significantly from one another. Not only does the average level of blood donation vary across regimes, the composition of the donor pool does as well. Individual characteristics have the same broad effects on the odds that a person will ever have given blood as they did in the country-by-country analyses, but the collection regimes change the magnitude of these effects in significant ways. While women in state regimes are about 65 percent as likely as men to have ever donated, this gap is about half as large again in blood-banking regimes. Red Cross countries also have a wider gender gap than state regimes, though to a lesser degree. In state regimes, moving up an income group raises the odds of having given by about 10 percent, while in Red Cross regimes this relationship, though significant, is flatter; increasing income raises the odds of having given by less than half as much.

Figure 4.3 shows how collection regimes change the effects of some individual characteristics on the probability of donation. The first panel shows that the effect of additional years of education, while always positive, is larger under state regimes than either of the alternatives. State regimes have more donors on average and are also more likely to have more educated donors. The second panel shows the strong contrast in the effect of ties to transfusion recipients between state and Red Cross regimes. In state regimes, as with education, each additional tie raises the probability of donation. But in this case, Red Cross regimes take advantage of additional ties to a significantly greater degree. A person with two or more ties living under a Red Cross regime is more likely to have donated than a comparable individual in a state regime. The difference does not lie in their individual character but in the structure of the collection system that provides them with opportunities to donate.

We see a similar effect for students. In state regimes, students are significantly less likely than average to have given blood. The effect is the same in blood-banking countries. But in Red Cross countries this effect is dampened: students are much more likely to have given blood than in other regimes. Again, this strongly suggests that the recruitment and retention strategies of collection organizations have a decisive effect on the kind of people who are likely to have given blood.

This comparison of collection regimes suggests that state and Red Cross countries are distinctively different from one another, with blood-banking regimes showing more internal heterogeneity. In particular,

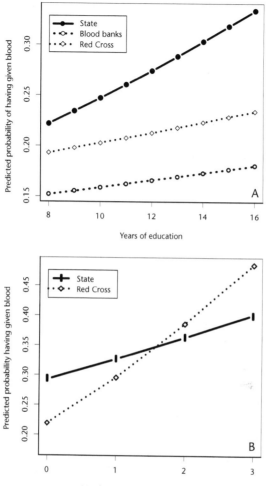

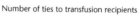

Figure 4.3. How collection regimes change the effect of individual characteristics on donation. Panel *A* shows that increasing years of education always increases the odds of having given blood, but the size of the effect varies with the collection regime. Panel *B* shows that having more ties to transfusion recipients increases the odds of having given blood, but more so in Red Cross than in state regimes.

while in state regimes being older, better-educated, and wealthier all make you more likely to have ever given blood, in Red Cross regimes these characteristics make less of a difference. In state systems being a student makes you much less likely to be a donor; again this effect is almost canceled out in Red Cross systems. Knowing someone who has received a transfusion is much more important in Red Cross systems than in state systems. Red Cross regimes recruit via these connections more effectively than do state systems. The mechanism might be quite general (such as appealing to recipients to tell their friends to donate) or it might be a more specific part of the donation process (such as strongly encouraging potential recipients to have a relative come in and donate blood for them).

The presence of donor organizations is the other main feature of the institutional environment. Respondents in the survey are more than twice as likely to have ever donated if they live in a country with a volunteer donor organization. Donor groups shift the effect of some individual characteristics in modest ways, perhaps flattening the positive effect of age and income on donation. But in general they do not strongly change a country's donor profile even though they significantly increase the size of its donor pool.

Finally, what about the effects of a commercial plasma supply? The claim that such enterprises tend to suppress voluntary donation is difficult to test given the data, but there is some support for it. We have seen that income has a broadly positive effect on donation. If we look at people in the bottom quartile of the income distribution, we find that they are generally less likely to donate blood than those with higher incomes, though this is not true in all countries. (Low income does not make a difference either way in Belgium, the Netherlands, and Italy.) In Spain and Germany, the two countries where it is possible to sell one's plasma, this effect is larger than average. Having the opportunity to sell plasma may reduce one's likelihood of giving blood. However, the data do not allow us to say conclusively whether opportunity to sell plasma is the reason that the poor are somewhat less likely to give. It seems unlikely to be the main reason. Only a very small percentage of people have ever given plasma, and the available information does not allow us to distinguish between those who sold it and those who donated it.

———

We think of blood donation as an exemplary act of altruism. What could be more selfless than giving away one's own blood to a stranger in need? Yet it is an odd kind of gift, for it cannot be given away as we might hand money to a needy stranger. In a way, this only increases the altruistic significance of donation, as it means donors cannot know or be thanked by those who receive their blood. But it also makes blood collection an organizational problem rather than an individual action. With the exception of Titmuss's pioneering effort of thirty years ago, the role of institutions in producing volunteer donors has not been studied comparatively.

This chapter outlined the range of organizational variation in European blood collection and showed its effects on donation. State-run systems have a larger than average donor base, concentrated in a male population of relatively high socioeconomic status. Countries with Red Cross systems, by contrast, tend to have fewer donors, and educational attainment and income have less of a positive effect on the odds of donation. Knowing transfusion recipients makes a big difference in Red Cross countries. Countries with blood-banking systems show the widest range of variation in donation rates. Volunteer donor groups increase the size of the donor pool but without greatly shifting its composition.

The analysis also revealed that having a different type of collection regime does not simply increase or decrease the donation rate along a sliding scale. Rather, it shapes the kind of activity that blood donation is. The analysis suggests that under a state regime, blood donation is something that people are likely to do once or twice, perhaps during a large collection effort. Under a Red Cross regime, blood donors are much more likely to be recruited through network, and especially family, ties when blood is needed. State systems pick up donors more extensively but do not retain them as successfully. Nor do they tap into the potential relationship between blood donation and other forms of volunteering. Blood-banking systems vary more, with those in southern Europe differing from those in northern Europe. The gender gap in donation is widest in blood-banking regimes in southern Europe. Denmark and Norway also show the highest ratio of regular donors to the overall donor pool, whereas other countries with blood-banking systems have relatively lower proportions of regular donors.

A comparative analysis at this cross-national level does not allow us to delve in detail into the organizational practices that produce the differences we observe between collection regimes. We should also bear in mind that there are other sources of variation that we cannot address within this framework—regional differences within countries, for example, or variability due to differences between organizations within the same country, of the sort analyzed in chapter 3.[29] Nevertheless, we can see that how you organize a blood supply system not only affects how much you collect and who you get it from, it shapes the character of donation. Collection regimes can make blood donation work like other forms of giving or make it quite unlikely that a donor will give more than once. Individuals may be moved to give their blood for any number of reasons, but it is the social organization of donation that offers individuals the chance to donate in the first place. Collection regimes embed altruism by creating opportunities to give. In the process, they produce differing donor populations. There is more than one way for a society to depend on the kindness of strangers.

FIVE

Organizations and Obligations

The argument so far has highlighted the role of organizations in the exchange of blood and organs. I have shown that we cannot understand why individual donors give without understanding the way collection organizations provide them with opportunities to donate. As we have seen, the efforts of collection organizations encompass both short-term logistical activities and long-term cultural work. The different ways they approach the problem of procurement leads to variation in the volume and sources of the supply of human goods.

This emphasis might lead us to think of these organizations as purely strategic entities. They feed donors plausible-sounding stories about why giving is a good thing to do, herd them into pens, and collect the products they need. In this picture, collection organizations are like puppeteers, cleverly manipulating donors but remaining immune to the accounts of altruism they themselves produce. In fact, these organizations do not stand outside the system of exchange manipulating the participants. Rather, they constitute the system and are themselves engaged in a social relationship with the donors and recipients. Instead of simply deploying their account of donation in a narrowly strategic way, they come to identify themselves as occupying a role with particular obligations to the other parties in the system.

This takes our general argument about the role of organizations in exchange a step further. In earlier chapters, we have seen how the distinctive features of the gift relationship—its Maussian dimensions of inalienability, obligation, and relatedness—structure the meaning of exchanges for donors. Collection organizations produce and reinforce their account of the gift, but they are not immune to its content. Once they become institutionalized, systems of exchange do more than just frame motives and provide opportunities to individual donors. They also embed the collection organizations themselves in ongoing relationships with suppliers and recipients. Over time, this will affect how staff in the organizations perceive their environment and make decisions. They may come to think of their loyalties as lying with one group rather than another, for instance, or react to changes in a way conditioned on the nature of their ties to different exchange partners. Just as individual donors and recipients have views about the content and consequences of the gift relationship, so too will the collection organizations that facilitate it. This can have important consequences when the broader environment changes unexpectedly.

In this chapter, I illustrate this argument through a study of the response of different organizations involved with the blood supply to the emergence of human immunodeficiency virus (HIV). In the early 1980s blood suppliers in most Western nations went through at least a crisis, in many cases a scandal. Thousands of people were infected with HIV after receiving blood transfusions or some other blood product. Blood-borne AIDS, like the AIDS epidemic as a whole, was a human tragedy. It was also an organizational disaster. The experience of the United States provides a particularly important starting point. It has the largest blood industry in the world and is unusual in that a nonprofit whole-blood sector that relies on voluntary donations coexists with a large, for-profit plasma industry that buys its raw material from suppliers. The volume of raw plasma purchased each year is almost the same as the volume of whole blood donated. In retrospect, this division within the U.S. blood industry makes its operations a kind of natural experiment. Studying its responses to the HIV crisis between 1981 and 1983 will allow us to test and develop our ideas about the differing effects of market and altruistic forms of exchange on the safety of the blood supply, and the role of exchange relations and organizational structure on decision making.

The appearance of blood-borne AIDS was an instance of an awkward kind of uncertainty. Actors in the blood industry were not sure what was going on, and the available information was ambiguous. They constructed a set of standards—an "information order," in Carol Heimer's phrase—to evaluate the problem.[1] These standards were influenced by three factors: the *external dependencies* of these organizations, the *exchange relations* that bound them in different ways to their suppliers and recipients, and the *organizational ties* that linked them to other stakeholders in the blood industry. As we shall see, particular exchange relations—that is, how blood and plasma were transferred between suppliers, processors, and recipients—had an important effect on the outcomes. Narrowly economic interests and safety concerns were embedded in exchange relations that had a strong moral dimension, and these relations significantly affected how organizations acted.

Interestingly, Richard Titmuss's *The Gift Relationship* was partly responsible for the organization of the blood supply in the United States.[2] The book's message was so successful that many social scientists and the public generally still believe that the U.S. blood supply rests mainly on for-profit sales of whole blood, when this has not been the case for thirty years. In fact, the most notable practical effect of *The Gift Relationship* was that it prompted a reorganization of the U.S. system along voluntary lines. Changes in law and government policy encouraged people to donate their blood rather than offer it for sale. Accepting the arguments of *The Gift Relationship,* the U.S. government tried to ensure a clean and safe supply by removing the profit motive from the whole-blood business. However, the system's reaction to the appearance of AIDS between 1981 and 1983 shows that while Titmuss was right that the composition of the donor pool depended on the social relationship between suppliers and recipients, the link between the gift relationship and the quality of supply is subtler than he realized.

Titmuss compared the social organization of the blood supply in England and the United States in the late 1960s and early 1970s. He argued that the then largely commercial, market-driven system of the United States was demonstrably inferior to England's voluntary system. In the United States, hepatitis was a chronic problem in the blood supply, whereas in England it was almost entirely absent. Titmuss claimed that if blood is a commodity, those who wish to sell theirs will have an incentive to lie about their health. Unsuitable suppliers will come forward and will be paid for a bad product. The people most likely to sell their blood are also those most likely to transmit disease. (Titmuss referred to them as "skid row" suppliers.) In addition to contaminating the supply, these commercial blood suppliers tend to drive volunteer donors away. By contrast, in an altruistic system there is no such incentive to lie; thus no one from "skid row" will donate blood and the supply will stay clean. In addition—and ultimately most importantly—altruism is morally better for society than the market. Markets are both inefficient and morally bankrupt. If blood remains a gift, then the system will stay efficient and the bonds of community will remain strong.

The Gift Relationship presents a strong mix of empirical facts and moral charges. The response to its argument was generally favorable at the time and has remained so. A few economists objected that Titmuss's argument underplayed the virtues of the market, but for once they were ignored.[3] In 1973, the Department of Health, Education, and Welfare announced the National Blood Policy, which recognized that reliance on "commercial sources of blood and blood components for transfusion therapy has contributed to a significantly disproportionate incidence of hepatitis, since such blood is often collected from sectors of society in which transmissible hepatitis is more prevalent."[4] The policy aimed to eliminate pernicious commercialism in the blood supply by instituting an all-volunteer system for the collection of whole blood.

From the perspective of economic sociology, Titmuss's book is an exemplary case of the "boundless model" of markets. The market is a voracious entity liable to eat up whatever it can get its hands on. Everything is in danger of becoming commodified, with the consequent destruction of social relationships and moral goods that cannot be measured in terms of money. The only defense against the market is the "legal preservation of selected items or activities outside of the cash nexus."[5] Some things— blood, for instance—should be kept sacred. Although motivated by a deep disgust with the market, this view nevertheless accepts that markets really are laws unto themselves, unbeholden to any social or cultural dampers.

Titmuss did not simply want to make a *moral* argument for the superiority of voluntary donation over for-profit sales. He thought that an altruistic system could beat the market at its own game. A gift-based system not only delivered a product that we could feel better about from an ethical point of view, he argued, but also one that was more efficiently obtained and of higher quality. The argument depended on two conditions being met. First, there had to be a clear way to link the organizational form of the collection system to the quality of the blood it procured. Some mechanism had to exist that ensured the one would affect the other. Second, this link would have to be unmediated by any other factors, so that the logic of the market and the logic of the gift could always be counted on to have their characteristic effects. Both of these assumptions were plausible when Titmuss made his argument, but it turns out that the link between a particular organizational form and a clean supply is contingent. More broadly, the form of the exchange relation is only one of several forces that impinge on the supply. It is not difficult to show the contingent nature of the connection between the form of the exchange and the quality of the supply. Understanding how the logic of gift and market exchange was mediated by other aspects of the organizational environment and the social structure will take us into a more detailed investigation of the HIV disaster.

Do Good Gifts Mean Clean Blood?

Titmuss was right to argue that, in the United States in the early 1970s, paying for blood tended to attract people who contaminated the supply. But he was wrong to suggest that contamination occurred because they were paid. Titmuss blurred the disctinction because he was mainly concerned with the hepatitis B virus (HBV). This was indeed prevalent among the supply population in the United States at the time. But this does not mean that we can assume that the price mechanism will always attract sellers with dirty blood.[6] Whether or not it does will be contingent upon the overlap of blood-selling and disease-bearing populations. Critics of Titmuss pointed out that some hospitals (like the Mayo Clinic) paid their suppliers and still managed to have a clean supply.

Consider. If there is a virus floating around in the blood supply that no one knows about, then how important is it whether people sell or freely give their blood to you? The answer is that, in the absence of epidemiological information, it is not important. More precisely, it may be true that market forms of organization attract infected populations. But the same might be said of voluntary forms. When the epidemiological profile of a disease is unknown, the extent to which either system appears to perform successfully is entirely dependent on whether the virus-bearing population is coextensive with its population of suppliers. To the extent that it is, the system will appear to be failing.

Titmuss wrote at a time when hepatitis was the main risk to the quality of the blood supply. Though recognized, this risk was not properly understood. "Serum hepatitis" (as it was then called) seemed resistant to attempts to weed it out of the system. There was no test that would reliably distinguish carriers from the general population. Tests existed, but they missed many carriers. It later turned out that this was because another virus, hepatitis C, was also being transmitted by transfusion.[7] Titmuss was lucky on both these counts. With one significant risk and no reliable test for it, he was able to assess the effectiveness of markets versus altruism as mechanisms for reducing that risk. The test of organizational efficiency was obvious: all one had to do was examine the prevalence of hepatitis among transfusion recipients. But this was an effective performance index only because of the unusual circumstances. Some of Titmuss's critics recognized this problem. They pointed out that the issue was not simply whether you paid for blood, but rather whether the person you paid had hepatitis.[8] If we had a different way to get information about supply quality—through epidemiology or accurate tests—then it wouldn't matter whether suppliers were paid or not, since we would not be relying on that mechanism to reduce the risk borne by the system.

Once we recognize that the relation between the social organization and the cleanliness of the supply is contingent, it is easy to see why neither voluntary nor price mechanisms can generally ensure anything about the quality of supply in cases where we do not know about a blood borne pathogen. Titmuss's argument about the beneficial effects of gift exchange on the quality of the supply is then greatly weakened. It amounts to saying that, when we know that a disease is chronic in the population we buy blood from, our blood supply will be dirtier than if we relied on voluntary donors who are less likely to have the disease. If a country has a naturally low rate of hepatitis across its population, or if a hospital carefully screens all its donors with a very reliable test for the disease, then it will not matter if the suppliers are gift givers or money-grubbers.

Both the United States and the European Union are at present committed to a volunteer-based blood supply, and Titmuss is properly cited as the inspiration in both cases.[9] But the terrible irony of *The Gift Relationship* is that its success helped create the conditions that allowed its argument to be turned upside down. In the case of HIV, the population of responsible, voluntary donors overlapped substantially with the disease-bearing population. Blood banks in large urban centers knew homosexual men to be reliable givers and good volunteers. As it turned out, they were also important vectors for HIV. The voluntary system ended up attracting people who contaminated the supply. But, as with commercial donors and hepatitis, the contamination happened not because they were donors but because they had HIV. The gift-based system ended up selecting the wrong people in much the same way that the previous market arrangement had selected the wrong people: by accident.

The connection between organizational form and supply quality is contingent, but that doesn't mean it's never observed. Diseases are socially distributed, usually in ways predictably related to income, class, or race. When Titmuss studied the supply, it really was the case that a blood-borne disease was much more prevalent among people likely to sell their blood. In this respect, his book had an important and beneficial effect. Indeed, to be fair to *The Gift Relationship*, these distributions would probably lead us to expect "Titmuss effects" more often than not. In general, the better-off are both less prone to illness and more likely to be blood donors. Therefore supply arrangements that select for the former will also happen to select for the latter. But like most useful rules of thumb, this assumes that important underlying conditions will not change over time. It is dangerous to ignore the potential for uncertainty. The U.S. blood supply managed to do so for about seven years. Then something new showed up and the system failed to deal with it.

To understand what happened to the supply in the early 1980s, we need a better theory. I argue that organizational responses to the emergence of HIV are best understood as a process of risk management operating under social-structural constraints. When a new uncertainty arises, these constraints provide the grid within which a response will be formulated. In 1981, the relative importance of suppliers and recipients, and the kind of exchange relationships they had with one another, gave managers a set of reference points that guided them as they evaluated new information and made decisions.

The U.S. Blood Supply

Getting blood or plasma out of one person and safely into another is a complicated business, and at present the people of the United States have two different kinds of organizations to do this job for them. First, there are blood banks (including the Red Cross), which obtain almost all of their supply from voluntary donors.[10] They process and then distribute freely donated blood. They charge hospitals for their services but are nonprofit organizations. Every year in the United States about fourteen million units of blood are donated to these organizations. In 1995 the American Red Cross collected about 45 percent of the total, community blood banks about 42 percent, and hospitals 11 per cent, and the small remainder was imported.[11] These donations are processed into different blood products: whole blood, plasma, clotting factors, and others. About 3.6 million people receive transfusions of these products every year. Blood banks generally enjoy local (geographical) monopolies. They do not compete with one another.

Plasma companies are the second kind of organization. They pay people to undergo plasmapheresis. A supplier is paid about fifteen to twenty-five dollars for a somewhat uncomfortable hour or so, during which about seven hundred milliliters of the liquid portion of his or her blood is extracted and the red cells are returned to the body. It is estimated that about thirteen million units of plasma are purchased in the United States each year.[12] There are four U.S.-based companies. These organizations process plasma and sell it to those people who need it—mainly hemophiliacs. There is a competitive market for plasma products.

In 1981 neither the blood banks nor the plasma companies were in any danger of being sued for infecting their recipients. "Blood shield" laws passed in the 1950s and 1960s exempted blood and blood products from strict liability or implied warranty claims, on the basis that their transfer was a service rather than a sale. The collective benefits of having a blood supply overrode individual rights to damages. A test case in 1977 confirmed that the plasma companies were covered by these laws in the same way as the blood banks.[13]

It would be highly impractical for an individual to negotiate a blood transfusion for herself. Individuals do not have the time, money, or expertise to obtain blood and monitor its quality. They must rely on these organizations to do it for them. Just as with organ donation, blood collection organizations promote an ideal image of the gift relationship between donors and recipients that overlies the logistical work done by a complex organization. The main challenge facing organ procurement organizations is the location and recovery of donors under tough time constraints. The organizations in charge of the blood supply must find donors and also minimize the danger that donors or (especially) recipients will become infected as a result of contaminated blood.

When there is good information about risks, this process is reasonably straightforward. Most blood is processed and delivered safely. Difficulties arise when unexpected events occur. In the 1970s, blood collection and transfusion had a number of risks associated with it, in particular the prevalence of hepatitis in the supply. But these problems were *risks* precisely because their probabilities were reasonably well known. In late 1982, when evidence began to show that a new disease might be spreading through blood products, things became more complicated. There appeared to be a threat, but its seriousness was difficult to measure. In such conditions, risk cannot easily be assessed. The blood industry was faced with real uncertainties about what was going on.[14] Nevertheless, these organizations were obliged to make decisions and act on the basis of the information they had. But although they were faced with the same uncertainties and armed with the same information, the blood banks and the plasma companies reacted in different ways.

In retrospect, the blood banks reacted badly: they played down the extent of the risk, they claimed that the evidence did not show conclusively that HIV was a blood-borne virus, and they refused to screen out potentially infected donors. By contrast, the plasma companies accepted that there was a good chance that HIV was being transmitted by their products, they moved very quickly to switch the source of their supply, and they introduced new methods to inactivate viruses in plasma derivatives. But these positive moves were mitigated by decisions to keep older batches of plasma products on the market, and in the end commercial plasma infected more people than did donated blood. Both the banks and the companies fell, albeit at different hurdles.

The Blood Industry's Information Order

There is a huge literature on the AIDS epidemic, but little of it deals directly with the blood industry. Relevant studies tend to fall into one of two categories: either they ignore the distinction between the commercial and noncommercial parts of the system or they tell the story in a whiggish way, with those who were in the right cast as heroes from the beginning.[15]

A richer theoretical perspective is available. In recent years, social scientists have paid increasing attention to the ways individuals and organizations manage risk and respond to disasters.[16] Of particular interest is the study of how organizations deal with uncertainty when doing so. When an organization knows the probability that some future event will occur, it deals in risk. Risks can be insured against or otherwise planned for. When future events are known to be possible but there is little or no information about the probabilities involved, an organization is simply uncertain about what is going to happen. To understand how structural interests, exchange relationships, and organizational ties shaped decisions within the blood industry, I draw on Carol Heimer's concept of a "negotiated information order."[17] Heimer studied how oil rigs in the Norwegian refining industry get insured. Drilling for oil in the North Sea is dangerous. In the late 1970s, it was a relatively new enterprise and so "experience-based information, usually the basis for decision making in marine insurance, was unavailable . . . there were no data about what the losses were likely to be."[18] To turn those uncertainties into insurable risks, the insurers and drillers developed a set of standards and routines for evaluating the information they had. Heimer points out that the going standard for knowing that something is true varies with the institutional setting: "When several actors are required to carry out [a] decision, then the problem is not so much to get evidence to answer the question, but to get information that everyone concerned will agree is evidence. That is, the information needs to be socially sufficient as well as technically sufficient."[19] The negotiated information order is the set of criteria for the social sufficiency of information. It is partly determined by the interests and bargaining power of the participating organizations.

Heimer's refiners and insurers had a well-worked-out set of rules, a stable information order. This was partly because they were oriented toward solving the problem of insurance from the beginning. In the case of the blood supply, the blood banks and plasma companies had to negotiate an information order on the fly, as they gradually became aware of the uncertainties they faced. The result was open conflict over the social sufficiency of the data they had. As we shall see, some players could look at the available information about transfusion and AIDS and say, "How many more cases did they need?" whereas others just saw "iffy" cases and "soft and squiggly data."[20] The decision-making process—and the resulting information order—was shaped by the interests of those involved. It is not obvious what those interests were. What led the blood banks and plasma companies to act as they did? As noted above, three factors were decisive: the external dependencies of the major players, the exchange relations within which these dependencies were embedded, and the organizational ties that linked the industry to other interested groups.

As I have said, we can think of the blood banks and the plasma companies as organizations that mediate between suppliers and recipients of blood and blood products, calculating risks and dealing with uncertainty as they go. When a problem like AIDS comes along the organization needs criteria to evaluate it. One option is to understand it in terms of its possible effects on suppliers and recipients. If there is a conflict of interest between these groups, an organization will move to protect the constituency it is externally dependent upon. Social-structural relations of relative power and dependency condition the interests of the organization, and valuable or important relations will be better attended to.[21]

The blood banks and plasma companies had different dependencies. For the banks, suppliers were relatively more valuable than recipients. Given a choice, blood bankers would much rather have a new supplier than a new transfusion recipient. Suppliers are relatively rare. Recipients are all too common. Given the same choice, plasma companies would much rather have a new recipient than a new supplier. In cases where the organization is caught in a conflict of interest between suppliers and recipients, it will tend to side with the constituency most valuable to it. The blood banks had a hard time finding and keeping donors, but they had plenty of recipients for these gifts. The plasma companies had a more or less stable population of recipients—determined in part by largely uncontrollable factors like the prevalence of hemophilia—that was much smaller than the population of potential suppliers. Their interests pointed to different constituencies.

The idea of external dependence is a useful way to grasp the structural basis of organizational interests. In this case, the exchange relationships that linked organizations to their suppliers and recipients influenced their actions independently of their interests. The external dependencies were embedded in a set of norms and expectations of exchange that either dampened or exacerbated them. In the case of blood donation, organizations structurally dependent upon suppliers obtained units of blood as voluntary gifts. By contrast, plasma organizations, structurally dependent upon recipients, contracted with their suppliers and sold their products in a competitive market. The social obligation of the blood banks to their suppliers reinforced their dependency. Making blood a gift tends to sacralize it, placing the receiver in a relationship of gratitude to the supplier. The Red Cross had drawn on this powerful trope of gift giving for years, in an effort to create a moral community of devoted givers, and after 1974 the blood banks joined them. The gift relationship made it very difficult for the blood banks to treat their suppliers in certain ways. In particular, it made the banks reluctant to reject blood or directly question its quality. No such bonds existed between the plasma companies and their suppliers or recipients. In the case of plasmapheresis, contract and payment define and discharge the obligations of the transaction, leaving all parties free of further responsibilities.

The consequences of each organization's structural dependencies were channeled through the exchange relations it had with suppliers and recipients. This is an important part of what it means to say economic interests and actions are socially embedded.[22] Suppliers can merely be suppliers, or they can be donors. Recipients can be patients or customers. When it comes to understanding why particular decisions were made, the structural dependencies and the exchange relations are analytically separable from one another and have independent effects.

If we did not make this distinction, we might think that the blood banks' supply pool was small simply because they did not pay for blood, whereas the reverse was true for plasma companies. This is incorrect, for two reasons. First, we are concerned here with the relative importance of the supply and demand populations in each case, not their absolute size. In absolute terms, more people donate blood than are paid for plasma. Second, imagine that only a tiny percentage of the population were physically able to donate plasma, whereas a large number of people actually needed it. (This might be true locally in times of war or after a natural disaster, for example.) In this case plasma delivery organizations would be externally dependent upon suppliers regardless of whether they paid those who showed up at the hospitals. Conversely, if donating blood was very easy and not many people needed it very often, then even a nonprofit organization would be more dependent upon recipients than suppliers for its survival.[23] The blood banks and plasma companies were externally dependent on their respective suppliers and recipients. This dependency defined their interests, but was itself embedded in a social relationship—either gift giving or market pricing. The structural and the social relationship were closely related, and variation in the one would most likely affect the other. But they were distinct, and need not have pushed in the same direction.

Finally, the blood banks and plasma companies were themselves situated in important relationships with other organizations. These include government agencies, health authorities, the medical profession, and groups representing suppliers and recipients. In each case, the kind of relationship that exists will affect how the organization interprets new information. I will focus on two organizations that significantly affected responses in each case. The blood banks' decisions were influenced by their relationships with gay rights groups and with the Centers for Disease Control, which is responsible for monitoring mortality and morbidity in the United States. Links to the medical profession and the National Hemophilia Foundation were both important in the case of the plasma companies. In the former case, the blood banks' attitude toward gay rights groups and the CDC tended to encourage the conservative and defensive stance they were already inclined to take. In the latter, the initially positive response of the plasma companies tended to be significantly watered down by the mediating influence of physicians and the NHF.[24]

The Blood Banks: Defending Suppliers

This was how things stood in 1981. In the case of nonprofit blood banks with voluntary donors, recipients bore the risk of receiving dirty blood. The recipient trusted the bank to minimize that risk, but the bank bore no liability for passing contaminated products to the recipient. The law said blood was a service, not a product, and the banks could not be sued for supplying bad blood. Strictly speaking, the supplier bore no risk either. Blood is a gift that is safe to donate, and donors are not culpable for any poisoned gifts they may hand over. Of course, the blood banks had no interest in actually killing their recipients, so they tried to ensure a safe supply. There was a problem with transfusion hepatitis, which was controllable but could not be eliminated. The banks were both externally dependent upon their donors and obliged to them for their gift. Only about 8 percent of eligible donors give blood in any one year, and the number of regular donors is much smaller still.[25] The gay community was known to be a good source of donors, having been drawn into the system in the 1970s during the effort to develop a vaccine for hepatitis B.[26] (Hepatitis was endemic in the gay population at this time.) This meant that, in the case of the blood banks, the risk bearers (recipients of transfusions) were different from the people the blood banks were obliged to and reliant upon (blood donors). This imbalance had serious consequences for recipients.

If they are to deal with uncertainty at all, organizations need information about what is happening. There are two important facts about the flow of information in the case of the HIV crisis. First, we know what information was available at various times during the disaster. Second, we also know that all the organizations involved got this information at the same time—and often at the same meetings. This means we can be sure that differences in response were not simply the result of some organizations' being better than others at gathering news. Rather, organizations processed the same information in different ways—why there were differences is what needs to be explained. This is also true for outcomes: the information base *was* the same and (in retrospect) the decisions made by the blood banks and the plasma companies *ought* to have been about the same. Thus, our attention is focused on the reasons why the decision processes within each set of organizations produced different outcomes.

Evidence of blood-borne AIDS transmission began to appear in December 1981.[27] A small number of hemophiliacs were found to have the same sort of immune-suppressive disorder that had been seen in homosexuals and recent Haitian immigrants. By August or September of 1982, epidemiologists at the Centers for Disease Control were sufficiently convinced that people were being infected by transfusions to suggest that blood banks not accept high-risk donors. In December 1982, the first fully documented case of AIDS transmission by transfusion was reported. Bruce Evatt, an epidemiologist with the CDC, began to present the data he had collected to various interested parties, including the Blood Products Advisory Committee (BPAC) of the Food and Drug Administration. On January 4, 1983, the CDC held a public meeting at its headquarters in Atlanta. Representatives attended from the FDA, NHF, the National Institutes of Health, the National Gay Task Force, plasma fractionators, and blood suppliers.

At the meeting, Evatt and James Curran presented their data and conclusions about the new disease and made a number of recommendations. Evatt had data on seven cases of AIDS in which it seemed that the victims (for example, small children) could only have contracted the disease through blood transfusions. On the basis of these cases, the CDC recommended that blood banks and plasma fractionators screen out homosexual donors and implement a surrogate test for the virus they believed must be the cause of AIDS.[28]

The organizations involved now had to decide what to do with this information. When asked about it during a 1994 investigation, those who attended turned out to have widely differing recollections of how the meeting was conducted, the effectiveness of Evatt's presentation, and the strength of his data. Evatt himself remembers being "stunned and depressed" by the response he received.[29] The epidemiologists saw the beginnings of a exponential growth curve and expected the number of new cases of the disease to rise rapidly. As can be seen from figure 5.1, this was the correct interpretation. At the time, however, opinions differed on the right way to read the data.

Blood bank representatives reacted by denying that the evidence was conclusive. Dr. Aaron Kellner, president of the New York Blood Center, said, "There are at most three cases of AIDS from blood donation and the evidence on two of these cases is very soft."[30] A program of donor screening would cost money, and false positives would mean that a lot of good blood would be thrown away. Dr. Joseph Bove, director of the blood bank at Yale University Hospitals and chair of the FDA committee on blood safety, said, "We are contemplating all these wide-ranging measures because one baby got AIDS after a transfusion from someone who later came down with AIDS and there may be a few other cases."[31] Later, blood bankers admitted that there was a risk of contracting AIDS through a transfusion but claimed that it was less than one in a million.

Claims about the likelihood of contracting AIDS through transfusion were not based on statistical risk assessment in any formal sense. The data were not good enough to do this kind of analysis. In an interview in 1994, Jay Epstein of the FDA noted that, in retrospect, those who thought the objective risk was low had "no scientific basis for that belief. . . . Instead of operating under the assumption of an unknown risk, they operated under a low risk assumption." Dr. June Osborn also attended the January 4, 1983, meeting. She noted in her 1994 interview that she did not believe a formal model of cost versus risk was formulated until after 1985, when the ELISA test for HIV came into use.[32] Although the vocabulary was the same, the language of risk was socially rather than technically grounded. Mary

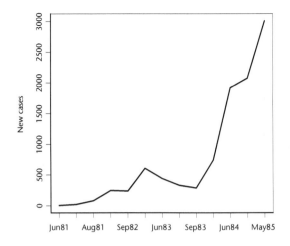

Figure 5.1. Reported cases of opportunistic infections and AIDS in the United States, June 1981–May 1985
Note: Data from IOM, *HIV and the Blood Supply.*

Douglas has made this argument in her work on risk and culture. As she suggests, phrases like "benefits and risks" were used by the blood industry "in an antique mode . . . to legitimate policy or discredit it." Douglas argues that "the neutral vocabulary of risk is all we have for making a bridge between the known facts of the world and the construction of a moral community."[33]

Later in January 1983, the blood banks issued a statement saying they did not want to ask people about high-risk sexual practices. They had ethical objections to limiting voluntary donation from high-risk groups, saying that "direct or indirect questions about a donor's sexual preference are inappropriate."[34] They did encourage autologous donations, especially in advance of elective surgery.[35]

The overriding reaction, as we would expect, was to deny that there was a problem with the supply. The January statement stressed that "the possibility of blood borne transmission [was] still unproven."[36] In private, the banks were more forthright in their opposition. The banks later added questions about AIDS symptoms to their standard list of questions before donation. However, they continued to oppose directly questioning donors about their sexual behavior, and neither did they recommend surrogate testing. An internal American Red Cross memo circulated in February 1983 indicates how officials in the voluntary sector were thinking at this time:

Relevant facts are: (1) the focal group of concern is the gays, we are not likely to incur much resistance with respect to elimination of any other group; . . . (3) homosexuals and bisexuals constitute up to 25 percent of the donor population . . . [male homosexuals] probably equal 15 percent or less of the donor population; . . . the scientific basis for elimination of gays [from the donor pool] does not exist at present.[37]

Blood banks' refusal to test for coindicators of AIDS indicates that they were reluctant to take the time and money to question the quality of the gift that was being given them. External dependence on their suppliers meant that they were particularly aware of the implications of screening out homosexuals. The well-organized gay rights lobby saw the question as one of personal autonomy. It argued that the evidence did not warrant what would amount to outright discrimination against homosexuals. The blood banks tended to agree. The author of the same memo says, "Ethically, I don't think sexual preference is the proper business of anyone (or any institution)."[38] This kind of concern from the blood banks was confined to homosexuals, however. Groups with no representative organizations were more easily removed from the donor pool, although even this took some time. Prisoners and Haitians were excluded on the grounds that they had a high rate of hepatitis, which was the most reliable surrogate marker for AIDS at the time. Male homosexuals had a higher rate of HBV than members of either of these groups but were not excluded.

The blood banks began with the view that a volunteer blood donor is an altruistic person who, despite the inconvenience, takes the time to donate blood. The idea of confronting such a donor with a prying and personal question about his sexual behavior seemed reprehensible and potentially very damaging to donor motivation. . . . In addition, the blood banks perceived that the gay community might not co-operate if gay donors were rejected on the basis of sexual orientation and, furthermore, that they might donate on purpose out of spite.[39]

Relationships with other organizations in their environment also influenced the way the blood banks evaluated the available evidence. These other groups had their own interests, which might be to the detriment of the banks and their donors. The American Red Cross's own analysis of the motives of the CDC (in an internal memo from January 1983) is particularly striking:

Even if the evolving evidence of an epidemic wanes CDC is likely to continue to play up AIDS—it has long been noted that CDC increasingly needs a major epidemic to justify its existence. This is especially true in the light of Federal funding cuts. . . . In short, we can *not* depend on CDC to provide scientific, objective, unbias [*sic*] leadership on the topic. However, because CDC will continue to push for more action from the blood banking community, the public will believe there is a scientific basis and means for eliminating gays.[40]

Similarly, at a meeting of the Blood Products Advisory Committee in February 1983, the participants heard a summary of the cases of transfusion AIDS that the CDC had identified. This evidence was given by Dennis Donohue, the director of the FDA's Division of Blood and Blood Products. Donohue described the case reports as "very soft and squiggly data."[41] When asked whether the cases were accepted as valid evidence by the CDC, Joseph Bove (the committee chairperson) responded, "Yes. Oh, my goodness, they are hanging everybody on the basis of it. . . . [These cases] are all, you know, very iffy."[42] In his interview with the Institute of Medicine committee in 1994, Bove said he "wanted to see the relationship between the transfusion patient and AIDS proven to be closer cause and effect [*sic*]—that the recipient had no other risk factors and that the donor came down with the disease; and that the donor gave twice and both the recipients came down with AIDS. Now I know I was asking for too much. But the epidemiologic data were not good in 1983."[43] The banks' assessment of risk was strongly conditioned by existing, institutionalized relationships with suppliers and other organizations. Their attitude was that if you looked a gift horse in the mouth, not only were you being churlish, you risked having your nose bitten as well. The blood banks chose to play down the problem and defend their suppliers' interests as their own. Unwilling to violate or question the gift relationship that gave them their blood, they acted as if reaffirming their trust in donors was the same thing as reducing the risk borne by recipients.

The Plasma Companies: Defending Recipients

As was the case with blood, plasma recipients bore the risk of exchange and trusted the companies to minimize it. The same liability laws applied. But in this case, the risk bearers were the more valuable group from the organizations' point of view. The market for plasma was competitive, and consumers might easily have bought a competitor's alternative. The plasma companies also had an interest in keeping their suppliers, of course, but this was largely solved by paying them for their time and effort.

The plasma companies had the same information available to them as the blood banks, were in the same legal position, and were faced with much the same range of choices. They reacted differently. Starting in December 1982, Alpha Theraputics began questioning donors directly. It excluded Haitians, homosexual males, and intravenous drug users from its supply population. A memo circulated to its affiliates identified the relevant risk groups and ordered them excluded from the company's supply population. The memo said, "While we recognize the potential for the rejection of long term donors, we strongly believe that the loss of these donors is more than offset by the protection of our patients."[44] This move was strongly opposed by the gay community and the blood banks. The former protested that they were being unfairly discriminated against; the latter knew that gay men were a major source of the blood supply in many urban areas and wanted the blood industry as a whole to have a consistent approach to the issue. The plasma companies, which had no moral commitment to their suppliers, ignored this opposition.

After the January 1983 meeting in Atlanta, the American Blood Resources Organization, the representative body of the plasma companies, issued recommendations about donor screening and deferral to reduce the risk of AIDS. In addition, news of AIDS in the blood supply caused research into viral inactivation methods to be accelerated. All of the U.S. plasma fractionators applied to the FDA to license treatment methods between June 1982 and December 1983. All were producing heat- or detergent-treated antihemophilic factor (AHF) concentrate by February 1984.

Although the businesslike exchange relationships with suppliers and recipients initially pushed the plasma companies to protect their markets, more than half of the sixteen thousand or so hemophiliacs in the United States contracted AIDS from contaminated plasma products. There are a number of reasons for this. Research into ways to kill hepatitis viruses in AHF concentrate had begun in the 1970s but subsequently stalled. Plasma fractionators had the potential to develop viral inactivation methods prior to 1980 but failed to do so because most of the people they were selling their product to—hemophiliacs—were already HBV antibody-positive. The benefits of AHF concentrate were great, and their target population was already infected with a chronic but manageable disease. The plasma companies assumed that no further protection would be necessary: "Hepatitis was viewed as an acceptable risk for individuals with hemophilia because it was considered a medically manageable complication of a very effective treatment for hemophilia."[45]

In this case, the plasma fractionators fail on the same grounds as the blood banks. They had a set of known costs and benefits that they used to guide the marketing and further development of their products. But they assumed that HBV was the only virus in the plasma supply and that, because most of their customers had it, there was no need to develop a process to eliminate it from AHF concentrate supplies. They contrasted the large benefits brought by their products to the manageable cost of hepatitis, with the emphasis strongly on the benefits. When evidence about AIDS began to mount, the feeling in the industry was that, whatever this new problem was, its costs could not outweigh the benefits of antihemophilic factor and other related products.

At a BPAC meeting in December 1982, a representative of Cutter Biologics argued, "We need to keep the life-sustaining significance of this product to the patient, and the lack of clear-cut risk based on currently available information, foremost in our collective minds."[46] The anticipated arrival of an HBV vaccine had added to this reluctance (the first one became available in 1982), because uninfected people would be protected against it in that way rather than by some new manufacturing process. There were no market incentives to pursue the research. No one seemed to countenance the possibility that other serious pathogens or latent agents (like Creutzfeld-Jakob disease or HIV) might also be present in untreated AHF concentrate. Once AIDS appeared, the plasma companies were able to move quickly and in the right direction to defend their market, but by then most of the hemophiliacs were infected anyway.

The market mechanism also failed to deliver a safe product to recipients even when one became available. The plasma companies had reacted to the information by developing new, safer ways to manufacture AHF concentrate. By market logic, the new products should have had a distinct competitive advantage over the old. But aspects of the organizational environment deflected the effects of the market. Physicians were reluctant to prescribe the new product to their patients, despite its availability and greater safety. The Institute of Medicine reports that hemophiliacs who came to their doctors worried about catching AIDS from AHF concentrate were reassured in spite of the evidence.[47] Doctors were happy with the therapeutic effects of AHF, and that outweighed any other worries:

[P]hysicians tended to avoid, downplay, or deny the possible risk associated with the use of blood and blood products, one of the case studies revealed that physicians often responded to the initial questions of the patients with reassurances that the risk was not serious, that the patient was overreacting, that there are always risks, and that patients and doctors should wait and see what happens. . . . Physicians emphasized the known benefits of AHF concentrate and underweighed the risks of AIDS, which were still uncertain.[48]

The role of the plasma companies was further complicated by their relationship with the National Hemophilia Foundation. The NHF "served a crucial function as an intermediary between the sources of scientific and medical information (i.e., CDC, FDA, plasma fractionation industry) and the consumers of that information."[49] The foundation was funded in part by the plasma companies. The Institute of Medicine report concluded that "the NHF's credibility . . . was eventually seriously compromised by its financial connections to the plasma fractionation industry."[50]

In a series of newsletters, the NHF reassured both doctors and patients that they could safely continue treatment with older batches of AHF concentrate and other plasma derivatives that later turned out to have been infected. In July 1982 "Hemophilia Newsnotes" stressed that "it is important to note that at this time the risk of contracting this immuno-suppressive agent [AIDS] is *minimal*."[51] As with the blood banks, technically sufficient data to make this sort of statement about risk were not available.

The NHF took a conservative line throughout 1982 and 1983. Its Medical and Scientific Advisory Council (MASAC) did eventually recommend, at a meeting in October 1983, that blood products not be collected from homosexuals and members of other at-risk groups. But (like the plasma companies) the group continued to use the risk-benefit data they had regarding hepatitis as though it took care of uncertainty about AIDS. And like the plasma companies the NHF took the stance that the benefits plasma concentrates brought to hemophiliacs were just too large to be outweighed by information about a new disease. At worst, AIDS would probably be like hepatitis—endemic but manageable. At the October 1983 meeting, MASAC noted with approval that data from a CDC/NHF study showed the average life expectancy of hemophiliacs to have risen from eleven years in 1968 to twenty years in 1983. "These findings," the minutes noted, "put into good perspective the importance of the use of [plasma] concentrates vs the small risk of AIDS."[52] The NHF newsletter was still urging a conservative approach as late as January 1984. As a result of this reassurance, a variety of plasma products were kept on the market for longer than they should have been, and many more hemophiliacs contracted HIV than might otherwise have been the case.

The relationship of the plasma companies to their recipients was mediated by both the medical profession and the National Hemophilia Foundation. Both of these organizations underestimated the effects of AIDS. Doctor-patient and buyer-seller relationships were interdependent, and the representative bodies of the plasma companies and their recipients were also closely interwoven, in this case with negative effects.

With hindsight, there is no doubt that there was a right way and a wrong way to react to the information about AIDS that began to appear from June 1981. Decisions about donor screening, risk assessment, and patient treatment now all seem obvious. But the reactions of the blood banks and plasma companies cannot be rightly understood from this point of view. What hindsight grants us is accurate risk assessment, precisely what those involved did not have. What we can now see as risks were then simply uncertainties. Taking a risk means placing a bet, and in order to place a bet you must know the odds. From the point of view of the organizations involved at the time, bets had to be made but the odds were not obvious. In 1976, on the basis of three cases of swine flu, millions of Americans had been vaccinated. More people died from the vaccine than from the disease. The episode was a huge embarrassment for the government and the CDC, and it was fresh in the minds of the blood suppliers.[53] Had AIDS turned out to be a nondisaster like that, the blood banks would have appeared prudent and the companies foolish.

I have offered an explanation for why one set of organizations rather than another tended to do (what in retrospect turned out to be) the right thing, and why neither were entirely successful. In 1982 the blood banks and plasma companies found themselves living in a newly uncertain world as a potential crisis loomed. As the organizations tried to construct a viable information order, conflicts arose over the quality of data, the credibility of sources, and the standards for evaluation. This case was unusual in that what were needed were standards of evidence sufficient not to judge the riskiness of future projects but to establish the existence of an ongoing disaster. Decisions were shaped by structural interests, morally weighted exchange relationships, and interorganizational ties. External dependencies and the moral obligations built into gift and market exchanges combined to influence reactions to the new information. Blood banks were led to side with their suppliers and plasma companies with their recipients. This set of relationships was itself situated in an extended organizational environment that further affected how the banks and plasma companies behaved. Things might easily have been different. Had their external dependencies been different, the plasma companies might have moved to defend the wrong group. Had their ties to other organizations been different, the blood banks might have found it easier to get important information from their donors. Had their donors been paid suppliers, the banks might have found it easier to eliminate some of them from the supply pool.

Blood suppliers in other countries, particularly in Europe, faced similar uncertainties and obligations as they dealt with AIDS.[54] In the United States, the contrast between donors and sellers was key. But in countries with no paid suppliers, the Maussian aspect of donation remained important. Blood donation was a "total social fact," a practice that encapsulated and expressed the relationship of the individual to the community as a whole. In France, for example, the blood supply was generally thought to express the ideal of a moral community bound by "common blood."[55] It underpinned the organizational structure of the supply there and was one of the key considerations that prevented the government from using the (American) ELISA test for AIDS.[56] That decision led to widespread infection in the French supply pool and to the imprisonment of blood industry executives. Three government officials—former prime minister Laurent Fabius, social affairs minister Georgina Dufoix, and health minister Edmond Hervé—were also tried for manslaughter. The case was heard in March 1999. Fabius and Dufoix were acquitted. Hervé was convicted but given no sentence.

———

The reaction of the different segments of the blood supply to the same sequence of events were strongly influenced by the exchange relations between suppliers, collection organizations, and recipients. The structural dependencies of blood banks and plasma companies were embedded in altruistic and profit-seeking exchange relationships that were an important part of their identity. These, in turn, were set in the context of both wider organizational environments and cultural accounts of gift giving. Social obligations built into the exchange system strongly influenced how organizations negotiated standards of proof and set the criteria for a reasonable response to the unfolding crisis.

The gift relationship played a decisive role, but not in the way that Titmuss would have hoped. Titmuss was right to say that exchange relationships have important consequences for the blood supply. But, except contingently, they are not the mechanism by which good or bad blood is brought into the system. In a similar way to organ procurement organizations, the blood agencies favored an account of donation that emphasized the uniqueness and inalienability of the gift of blood. This entrenched, elaborated understanding of the meaning and significance of donation pushed the blood industry to react to new information in a counterproductive way. The implication is not that a market for blood is therefore superior. Indeed, as we have seen, the plasma companies and their allies also erred in their assessment of the risks because they were unwilling to stop using batches of untreated AHF concentrate. The HIV disaster does not tell us that we should unequivocally choose commodities over gifts. Rather, it brings out the interaction of both modes of exchange with the underlying organization of the supply, especially with the technical and manufacturing changes that have taken place since the publication of *The Gift Relationship.*

When Titmuss wrote, the gift of blood passed from giver to receiver in a fairly direct way, with little in the way of processing or refining in the intervening period. Today, blood is treated much more intensively to yield many derivative products with more specific uses and longer shelf lives. A donated unit may end up benefiting many more people, but the role of the intervening organizational layer is of necessity much larger and the connection between donors and recipients is less direct. The production of AHF from pooled donations was the earliest wave of this transformation. The HIV disaster accelerated as collection agencies implemented and publicized new methods of quality assurance, in order to allay public fear about the quality of the supply. They eventually tested every donation for potential contamination and systematically excluded segments of the population deemed too risky. These changes made the supply safer, though they did not fully allay the fears of donors or recipients.[57] As a result, it is now much more difficult for blood donation to generate solidarity in the way that Titmuss described. The industrialization of the supply brought with it a move from public trust in the institution of anonymous donation to uncertainty over the risk of participating in it.[58] As secondary markets in for human blood and tissues continue to grow, it is unclear whether the gift relationship, as presently understood, can continue to provide a plausible framework for the exchange of donor blood and body parts.

SIX

Managing Gifts, Making Markets

Here are three stories from the world of exchange in organs, blood, and tissue. In the autumn of 1999, Britain's Health Secretary launched an official inquiry into revelations that a number of children's hospitals had been removing organs from dead infants without the informed consent of their parents. As the inquiry progressed, other facts came to light. For a number of years, hospitals had routinely sold the thymus glands of live children to biotechnology companies (these glands are often removed during pediatric heart surgery). In cases where children died, their organs or other body parts had been removed. The organs were ostensibly collected for scientific research, but in fact they were simply bottled and stored. One of the largest such collections in the United Kingdom was at Alder Hey, a children's hospital in Liverpool. The inquiry's final report found that between 1995 and 1998 doctors at Alder Hey had systematically harvested all the organs of all the children who died at the hospital and underwent postmortem examinations there. The report blamed a hospital pathologist, Dick van Velzen, who failed to obtain consent from parents and lied to them about what was happening to their children's bodies. His colleagues and superiors at the hospital gradually became aware of his actions but failed to stop him.[1]

Although van Velzen was at the center of the scandal, the report made clear that he was continuing a tradition of organ and tissue collection at the hospital—and around the country—going back to the late 1940s. As of February 2000, Alder

Hey's collection included 2,124 hearts, 1,564 fetuses and stillbirths, 198 fetal eyes, 147 infant cerebella, and 22 major body parts from 15 children, including the head of an eleven-year-old boy. A Department of Health census of organ holdings in the whole of the United Kingdom counted more than fifty-four thousand organs and body parts being stored in hospitals around the country.[2] These findings provoked a national scandal. One effect has been a drop in the number of postmortems carried out. Doctors also feared that the number of organs being donated for transplant would decline.[3]

In the mid-1990s in Ireland, around a thousand Rh-negative women discovered that they had been infected with hepatitis C fifteen to twenty years before, when they had received contaminated anti-D immunoglobulin from the National Blood Transfusion Services Board while they were pregnant. The Irish government was very slow to respond to demands for an investigation, and it was only after protracted lobbying, and the death of one of the main activists, that a tribunal was convened to investigate the matter. Public confidence in the Irish blood supply was further damaged in the following years as official investigations into both hepatitis C and HIV contamination of the blood supply revealed a badly run and poorly managed service.[4]

Finally, in March 2004, the *New York Times* reported that the director of UCLA medical school's Willed Body Program had been arrested for illegally selling body parts from donated cadavers to medical research companies.[5] The program had previously been investigated in 1996 when it was sued by family members who alleged that the cremated remains of donated bodies had been mixed with medical waste and dumped at sea, rather than given a burial service as promised.[6] This was not the first time that stories like this had made the news. During the spring and summer of 2000, the *Orange County Register* and the *Chicago Tribune* each ran a series of stories on the market for human goods in the United States.[7] The articles focused on the trade in human tissue, a very broad category that includes everything that might be procured from a donor except the major organs. When donor families sign an organ donor consent form, they often agree to tissue procurement as well. Journalistic evidence suggests that families are sometimes unaware of the difference between the two. In particular, they do not realize that human tissue is traded in a secondary market made up of biotechnology, medical supply, and drug companies. One recent estimate suggested that the sale or trade of human goods from a fully processed donor could yield more than $222,000, though the average market value is closer to $80,000.[8] Some of the consumer markets for products derived from cadaver donors are not well known. For instance, skin

taken from donors is used to make Alloderm, a commercial product originally used to treat burn victims but increasingly in demand from cosmetic
surgeons, who use it in operations to remove facial wrinkles, reshape lips,
and enlarge penises. Partly in response to these stories, the federal Department of Health and Human Services investigated the tissue banking industry and found that it was not well regulated. More than 20 percent of
tissue banks had not been inspected in the previous five years.[9]

———

Alder Hey, anti-D, and Alloderm have all provoked strongly negative publicity: outrage on the part of the public, embarrassment on the part of the
authorities. Each case illuminates an aspect of the argument I have been
making. The response of the British public to the revelations about Alder
Hey shows that support for organ donation, and people's comfort with
the idea of organ harvesting, is fragile. Or rather, the public does not think
about these matters in the same way as the medical profession and the
human-goods industry. Most people living in Britain and the United
States have never seen a corpse. They support organ donation in the abstract, but the bureaucratized management of human tissue can easily
horrify them. This is to be expected when, as is alleged in the UCLA case,
organizations break their promises to donors. The Alder Hey inquiry ex-
posed tissue recovery and retention practices that were routine (and often
accompanied by signed consent forms) but which nevertheless appalled
the public. The recent scandals in Ireland show how trust in the blood collection and supply system can also easily be lost. As with HIV infection in
many other countries, the very ideals that blood suppliers depended upon
to keep donors rolling up their sleeves were well adapted to articulate the
outrage and betrayal felt by victims. The gift of life, the dignity of donation, and the rhetoric of community sit uneasily with the bureaucratic administration of procurement.[10]

These cases are also reminiscent of past scandals and disputes over
human goods. The outcry at tissue collection by hospitals and research facilities is similar to much older fears from the early days of transplantation
about out-of-control medical researchers. The hepatitis C infections were,
in many respects, a tragic recapitulation of the HIV disaster. Reports of
the burgeoning secondary market for human tissue read like the exposés
of blood selling in the early 1970s. Those stories provoked the last round
of serious debate about institutional design in this area, as public outrage
gave way to studies of how the system worked. Since then, the for-profit
use of donated body parts and products has increased dramatically, but

a sociology of the procurement system has not grown up alongside it. Anthropologists have examined the rapidly growing sphere of illegal or "gray" exchange, documenting the globalization of sales in kidneys and other organs, a market that depends on poor sellers in desperate circumstances.[11] In the United States, bioethicists and economists dominate public discussion of organ exchange in the formal economy. They have done important work on the ethics of informed consent and, more recently, the prospect of financial incentives for donation. But this has been accompanied by a narrowing of focus. Bioethicists, for instance, are attuned to questions of individual moral choice in medicine, and are less concerned with broader issues of social organization and institutional design.[12] Titmuss's work in *The Gift Relationship* should have led to the development of a systematic comparative sociology of exchange in blood and organs. But because of the book's immediate success in transforming American blood policy, its findings became a kind of "stylized fact," used anecdotally and in passing, but not subjected to further empirical testing or theoretical development. Titmuss was taken as saying that altruism is better than self-interest. His deeper argument about the relationship between social organization and individual action faded from view.

This book has challenged the image of the individual altruist who simply chooses, in the absence of organizationally managed opportunities or culturally sustained exchange relations, to come forward and do good. We have looked in detail at two paradigmatic cases of anonymous, altruistic giving and found that, in fact, they are moral economies sustained by procurement organizations. To reiterate: organizations produce donations by providing opportunities to give and sustain them by generating accounts of what giving means. Doing so entails a great deal of logistical and cultural work. It is variation in the degree and kind of this work that explains variability in collection rates. Collection regimes with different procurement strategies will produce distinctive donor populations with particular conceptions of what they are doing. Procurement organizations try to manage their suppliers, carefully but with varying degrees of success. This might suggest that organizations manage donors as ants tend to aphids, farming them assiduously and stroking them for nectar as needed. But individual expectations and organizational capacities have coevolved. Collection organizations become committed to their own public accounts of donation and think about their interests and obligations in ways that reflect the content of the relationship they have with suppliers and recipients. As was the case with HIV, this does not necessarily lead them to act in ways that benefit themselves or those they serve.

With these findings in mind, I want to conclude by discussing three broader questions. First, are our theories of the gift able to cope with exchange in human goods as we know it, given that body parts do not circulate like ordinary gifts and cannot in general be reciprocated? Second, will the gift exchange of human goods itself be caught between an increasingly industrialized procurement process and an inegalitarian, profit-driven medical system? And third, what are the prospects for market exchange in blood or organs? I will argue that established theories of gift exchange do not deal well with human goods; that the robustness of voluntary donation is an open question; and that the rationalization of procurement systems, together with the rise of lucrative markets in processed tissue, has prepared the way for commodification—but of a particular kind.

Self-Interest and Solidarity in Gift Exchange

In gift exchanges, people tend to avoid explicitly accounting for or discussing the economic value of their gifts, and yet they may also ensure that their gifts are reciprocated over a sequence of exchanges. This unacknowledged mutual monitoring can appear inordinately convoluted, especially if we admit the possibility that it is not just left publicly unacknowledged but is somehow not even admitted to oneself. It is difficult enough to give a good account of it for societies where gifts are the principal mode of exchange. The presence of markets makes the problem more complex. Pierre Bourdieu's approach is characteristic of the difficulties encountered when dealing with the enigmatic question of gift-based reciprocity across a whole society. Bourdieu does not want to reduce the act of gift giving to a simple exercise in accounting for one-to-one exchanges: that would make gifts too much like markets, and the gift giver too much like *Homo economicus*. But some sort of reckoning may take place, even if it is not acknowledged. So he argues that "practices always have double truths, which are difficult to hold together. Analysis must take note of this duality," which "is rendered possible, and viable, through a sort of *self-deception,* a veritable *collective misrecognition* inscribed in objective structures and in mental structures, excluding the possibility of thinking or acting otherwise."[13] How does this collective repression happen?

If agents can be at the same time mystifiers, of themselves and others, and mystified, it is because they have been immersed from childhood in a universe where gift exchange is socially *instituted* in dispositions and beliefs. Such exchange thus shares none of the paradoxes which emerge artificially when . . . one relies on the logic of consciousness and the free choice of an isolated individual.[14]

Bourdieu tries to smother the paradox by embracing it. The individual and collective repression of the purposive aspects of gifts is possible because it is part of the habitus, and so is a near-natural disposition of the body rather than a cognitive problem.[15] These dispositions are acquired through socialization. Individuals are "immersed from childhood" in the kind of society that exchanges gifts, so they come to act this way themselves.

This is an attractive but unsatisfactory view. Bourdieu explains the origin of the "collective misrecognition" by saying it is imparted through socialization and explains its persistence by saying that it is a noncognitive way of acting. But this cannot be the whole story because, as Bourdieu mentions himself, even strongly gift-based societies—like the Kabyle he studied in Algeria—have "numerous proverbs" pointing out that gifts can be demands in disguise. If they can articulate this paradox of gift giving, how can the society as a whole be collectively repressing it? We might say that there is a strong taboo, enforced in some way, on drawing attention to the calculating aspect of gift giving. Bourdieu acknowledges a "taboo of making things explicit" and a "taboo of calculation." This goes a little way toward a solution. We know that people are reluctant to be seen as too calculating in their actions, just as they are unwilling to be seen as too selfless. But Bourdieu does not simply want to say that people shy away from acknowledging the calculative aspect of gifts, but rather that people are in fact unaware that this aspect even exists. This also makes a second response unavailable to Bourdieu, the idea that individuals can draw on psychological tricks to ignore or repress something they really know. So he rejects the notion that "people deliberately close their eyes to this reality."[16] Intentionality has no place in his account, so none of the clever mechanisms for self-deception discussed by the likes of Jon Elster can apply.[17] Bourdieu finds this approach, which relies on the idea that the mind can be divided against itself, to be absurd. In the end, he provides no explanation for how this collective and individual self-deception is sustained.[18]

Having said that gift exchange is made possible via collective misrecognition supported by the habitus, and having denied that intentional action, individual strategy, and cognitive effort play any part in it, Bourdieu immediately makes an incisive observation about the role of euphemisms in gift exchange that does not sit well with his main argument. He describes one of the ways people deal with the calculative aspect of gift giving without fully expressing it:

Euphemisms permit the naming of the unnameable, that is, in an economy of symbolic goods, the economic, in the ordinary sense of the term, the exchange of exact equivalents. . . . There is no society that does not render homage to those who render homage to it in seeming to refuse the law of selfish interest. What is required is not that one do absolutely everything that one should, but rather that one at least give indications of trying to do so. Social agents are not expected to be perfectly in order, but rather to give visible signs that, if they can, they will respect the rules.[19]

This seems right. People use the "practical euphemisms" he describes in a way that produces the paradoxes associated with gift exchange. From Bourdieu's own description of this process, it is clear that it cannot help but be intentional to some degree, and understood by those who participate in the round of giving.

Gifts of blood and organs are a world away from kula rings and potlatch gatherings. Even if there were pure gifts in these systems, given freely with no expectation of return, there were no *anonymous* gifts. Anonymity would have undermined the particular social relationship affirmed by the exchange. But as we have repeatedly seen, despite the anonymity of exchange in human goods there is usually a strong concern that these gifts be treated in a manner appropriate to both giver and recipient. Cases where donor families feel their gift has been defiled bring this out very sharply, but it is also readily apparent in less controversial circumstances. Titmuss made this clear also. He knew that blood donors were not idealized altruists and also saw that they were not wholly anonymous. "None of the donors' answers was purely altruistic," he noted. "No donor type can be depicted in terms of complete, disinterested, spontaneous altruism. There must be some sense of obligation, approval and interest; some feeling of 'inclusion' in society; some awareness of need and the purposes of the gift."[20] It was the collection organization (in this case, the British National Health Service) that provided the link to the wider society and allowed donors to connect their personal reasons for giving with the general need for blood.

We saw in chapter 2 that organ donor families often think about the recipient of their gift.[21] They may imagine an idealized recipient, often one resembling the loved one they have lost. Similarly, the donors Titmuss surveyed often thought of specific people from their own pasts when they donated, or particular incidents they remembered as crystallizing the obligation to help. As a social practice, then, anonymous gift giving may incorporate personal elements that will be invisible in the exchange itself yet essential to its meaning. In her ethnographic study of volunteers at a charity that cooked meals for people with AIDS, Courtney Bender found these elements in the routine work of preparing food for anonymous recipients.[22] Like blood donors, the kitchen workers never saw the beneficiaries of their kindness, but—perhaps for this very reason—the volunteers often had some very specific ideas about them. These images of the recipients were often not shared by others at work in the kitchen, though many assumed they were. For Mauss, the reproduction of social solidarity through generosity, obligation, and repayment was accomplished through gifts circulating among specific, known individuals. Gift giving in modern societies often works this way within kin groups and small social networks. But there are many instances of anonymous gifts.[23] Blood and organ donors give of themselves with fictive recipients in mind. This imagined exchange is operationally managed and culturally elaborated by the procurement organization. It helps produce the social identities that make the exchange plausible.

How Robust Is the Gift Relationship?

Throughout this book, I have emphasized the vital role that organizations play in reproducing the gift exchange of blood and organs. As a matter of routine, they produce contexts in which people have the opportunity to give. Over the longer term, they also produce and institutionalize cultural resources—sets of ideas and stories, meant for public consumption, about the nature and meaning of what they are doing. This is what I have been calling the "cultural account of donation." These efforts are a severely neglected side of the gift relationship. Theories of the gift almost always center on the relationship between individual giver and individual recipient, with any mediating social organization either assumed away or underanalyzed. This flows from the anthropological origins of theories of the gift. The societies where gift exchange was first studied in detail required no organization to monitor compliance with the rules of giving or to intervene between givers and recipients to complete the transaction.

As we saw in chapter 2, the cultural account of donation is partly a set of principles, reasons, and examples meant to encourage support for donation. The arguments and principles are backed up (interwoven, rather) with examples and stories. Some of these are aimed at people who might want to sign a donor card; others describe the ideal set of feelings and reactions that people should have if they ever have to make the difficult decision to give up their next of kin's organs. These reasons, examples, and stories form a cohesive account that is prescriptive rather than descriptive and that presents a narrow set of ideal "feeling rules" rather than simply reflecting the varied emotional reactions people have to donation.[24]

In the United States, there are now almost ninety thousand people waiting for a transplant of some kind. Some of those will be given kidneys by living donors, and a tiny percentage will be given the lobe of a live donor's liver. But most will have to rely on a cadaveric donor being found. Fewer than seven thousand cadaver donors are procured each year. This structural pressure on the system has been building since the early 1990s and is now very severe. In the face of this constantly increasing demand, how robust can we expect the existing gift relationship to be? Is it just a flexible bit of marketing talk or is it more like an institutional logic that has been built in to the procurement system?[25] Public discourse about donation has already shifted as waiting lists have grown, with "market talk" about organs increasing rapidly since the late 1980s. Within the transplant industry, views about paying donors or donor families vary: surgeons are often bluntly in favor of any incentive system that increases the supply of organs and enables them to save people's lives. They are oriented downstream, toward the source of the demand. By contrast, procurement coordinators and OPO staff tend to be oriented upstream, toward the supply. They are more aware of the fluid nature of the consent process and more suspicious of financial incentives. In particular, they have long been wary of any proposal that might turn public opinion against organ donation in general.

The resilience of the cultural account of donation depends on whether—and to what degree—the staff of procurement organizations really subscribe to it. If they do, then it will be hard to dislodge it without damaging the procurement system, because these are the people who work directly to obtain consent from families. If their attitude is more ambivalent, then a relatively rapid reconfiguration of some sort may be more likely. The actual views of procurement staff in this respect is an open empirical question. At present, the "gift of life" account remains the dominant way that organ donation is publicly argued for. The transplant industry successfully overcame a queasy public's fears about transplantation by accounting for organ donation as a moral choice that created a special kind of relationship between donors and recipients. In a sense they are now victims of their own success: the public understanding of donation they created stands in the way of the introduction of financial incentives for organ procurement.

In addition to its internal strength, the future of gift exchange in human goods also depends on the likely effect of a market approach on the procurement rate. Commentators have tended to assume that the "give or sell" choice determines the ethical basis of a procurement system, usually through the effects of the transaction on the psychology of donors. This is typically how the options are presented in media coverage. But as we have seen, institutional and organizational differences both large and small can decisively affect procurement rates, independent of the general form of the exchange. On a large scale, all-volunteer systems of blood donation show substantial variation in the size and composition of their donor pools. On a smaller but no less important level, quite fine-grained organizational differences can have large effects on the organ procurement rate.

For example, our analysis of U.S. organ procurement organizations found that while a general willingness to pursue donors in difficult (but hypothetical) circumstances was not associated with increased procurement rates, key changes to procurement procedures did bring about significant increases in the procurement rate. The particulars mattered a great deal. Cases like that of South Carolina's LifePoint show that OPOs have the ability to change their logistical methods in order to increase consent rates.[26] LifePoint was restructured in a way that separated distinct procurement tasks into separate occupational roles. The position of family support counselor was created to help donor families cope with their time in the hospital and to inform them about brain death, while an aftercare coordinator arranged follow-up counseling and other support. Crucially, neither of these was responsible for requesting the consent of the donor family. Indeed, from the family's point of view, the support counselor who helped and informed them and the LifePoint coordinator who requested consent might not have been from the same organization at all.

They *were* from the same organization, of course. Organ procurement organizations must make sure that the next of kin give their informed consent, and this requires in part that the donor family not be deceived. Does the OPO's careful management of the procurement process meet this standard? The process is not that different from the practice of "cooling the mark out" described in a famous paper by Erving Goffman.[27] Here, a con artist and an associate carefully manage an interaction with their victim, or mark. Once the con has been concluded and the mark relieved of his money, the con artist sends in an associate who explains what has happened, commiserates with the mark, and reconciles him to his fate— perhaps even making him think it was his own fault. This "cooling out" period helps ensure that the mark doesn't report the crime to the police.

Now, organ procurement is not a con, but bioethicists worry that managing the consent process in an equally calculating way might make us unsure whether the consent of donor families is properly informed. Sociologically, however, this aspect of successful procurement is crucial. Effective OPOs must manage the consent process by breaking it up into its component elements, controlling the way in which the donor family gets information. Goffman's study is relevant because it emphasizes the way the fine structure of the interaction shapes the outcome and the feelings of the participants about what is happening, both during the procedure and especially afterward. Donor families are grieving, often in shock and sometimes confused. It is a mistake to think that, in such volatile circumstances, a decision is made after the pros and cons of the decision are dispassionately weighed in the light of one's preferences. It is in just such a case that clear information and guidance from a reliable source is needed, so that any choice is more than a reflex response one way or the other.

The relationship established by the OPO, and the time and personnel it invests in this relationship, is vital to both the needs of the families and the goal of the organization. The way the OPO manages the process is therefore inevitably strategic, but this does not make it immoral. A commitment to the principle of informed consent cannot by itself answer detailed questions about how the consent process should be managed: How much information does the donor family need to be given about the uses to which donated tissues might be put? Ought it be given all at once? What sort of language should it be presented in? As Onora O'Neill comments, a process that detailed everything would "bring the consent procedure into disrepute by reducing it to ticking boxes or signing paragraphs of unread fine print" and would "actually diminish trust by the very ways in which it seeks to demonstrate trustworthiness."[28] What separates procurement from Goffman's case, of course, is that donor families ought to be able to trust the OPOs to do the right thing, given that organ procurement is a routine event for them and they have far more knowledge about it than the donor family. However, there is nothing in either gift exchange or market exchange as such that can be relied on to automatically solve these problems of trust. Both forms of exchange have the potential to betray donors and recipients.

Commodification and Industrialization

Much of the work in economic sociology over the past twenty years has been devoted to challenging the paradigm of anonymous market exchange. The main target of this project has been neoclassical economics with its vision of disembodied, perfectly rational agents reaching stable equilibria under ideal conditions. Since the 1970s, economists have enriched the neoclassical model in an effort to incorporate imperfections in information, differences in institutional context, and asymmetries in power. But the dominant theme in that field remains the effort to reconcile these pervasive features of social life with the possibility of equilibrium states brought about by rational choices. Economic sociologists typically reject this picture, and with good reason. They often fail to see, however, that basic critiques of commodification are also undermined by their insistence on the embeddedness of economic action. The idea that markets inevitably corrupt is not tenable precisely *because* they are embedded within social relations, cultural categories, and institutional routines. It has taken some time for a view of markets to emerge that both develops Polanyi's idea that the economy is an "instituted process" and relaxes the claim that money and markets inevitably corrupt and undermine human relationships. The two ideas were often bound together by political conviction or moral intuition, as well as by evidence. The sharpest analyses of the social foundations of market institutions were often also the most powerful indictments of their effects.

We need to recast debates about commodification and altruism with this in mind. Rather than thinking of the willingness to give solely as a virtue found in some individuals and not in others, I have argued that it can be investigated in terms of its institutional underpinnings. Markets are no different, and the shared roots of our ideas about selfishness and altruism are underappreciated. To take a long view, the growth of commercial society in the seventeenth and eighteenth centuries brought the market and its potential effects to the forefront of social thought.[29] The growth and spread of market relations implied that there was a corresponding sphere of disinterested social association with no connection to commerce, and this gave birth to the modern concept of friendship for its own sake.[30] Experimental evidence bears out the link. In "ultimatum games," a person is given the opportunity to share a sum of money—say ten dollars, in units of one dollar—with someone else. The prospective recipient has to take or leave the offer that is made. If both parties acted purely as economic agents, the offerer would keep nine dollars for herself and the recipient would take the one dollar. After all, the offerer should rationally keep as much as possible and the recipient should see that a dollar is better than nothing. In fact, research repeatedly finds that offerers consistently make much fairer offers than this (perhaps keeping a small amount extra for themselves) and that recipients will reject lowball offers with contempt.[31] It is particularly striking, however, to learn that when these experiments have been performed in small nonmarket societies the results have generally not been replicated. The less experience the participants had with market exchange, the less likely they were to make generous offers. It appears that the prevalence of the market and a willingness to cooperate may go together: "The more frequently people experience market transactions, the more they will also experience abstract sharing principles concerning behaviors toward strangers. . . . The degree of cooperation, sharing and punishment exhibited . . . closely corresponds to templates for these behaviors in the subjects' daily lives."[32]

In contemporary societies, the complement of the idealized market transaction of commodities between two self-interested individuals is the notion of the present given freely and without any expectation of return—what Jonathan Parry has called "the elaborated ideology of the 'pure gift'."[33] Although useful markers of the ends of a continuum of exchange, neither of these ideals accurately reflects how market or gift exchanges typically take place. Either the gift or the sale of blood or organs establishes a particular social relation. As with many other exchanges, the parties need to be able to trust that the transaction will go as both intend. Usually it will be the donors who are most concerned about this, as the exchange may not be routine for them. Both gift-based and market-based forms have the capacity to secure the transaction to the satisfaction of all those involved. Both also have the potential to fail. The pitfalls of the market are perhaps easier to see: the seller may not get a good price or, worse, may feel that the attachment of a price to the transaction is an insult. The right form of payment may go a long way to securing confidence in the exchange: payment in kind or compensation for funeral expenses will be preferable to being handed an envelope of twenties in the hospital waiting room. Conversely, if donors are promised that their "gift of life" will be treated *as a gift,* then the discovery that it has been dumped, left unused, or sold at a large profit is likely to outrage them.

Regardless of whether they rely on financial incentives or goodwill, modern systems of procurement and exchange of human goods depend on complex organizations, which set the context for the exchange and establish the relationship with their suppliers. In most important respects, big, modern nonprofit corporations are closer kin to big, modern for-profit corporations than they are to small charitable groups run by volunteers. Whether exchange is commodified may matter less than whether it is *industrialized,* which is to say administered by rationalized organizations. Industrialized democracies and industrialized dictatorships look much the same to a society of hunter-gatherers. Rationalized organizational systems may look ruthless to people, and it is often their impersonal quality that provokes outrage. Both supporters of the market and critics of commodification miss this point when they think in terms of a sharp contrast between volunteers and profiteers.

For simple commodities, a sale means that the seller no longer has any claim to what is sold or say over what the buyer does with it. Similarly, under the elaborated ideology of the pure gift, it might seem strange or even hypocritical that people complain about the use to which their gifts are put. After all, they gave them freely, as presents. But on a Maussian view of exchange, it is not surprising that gifts can produce this reaction:

[It is not] that the giver always has the right to reclaim the object or that such a right could be exercised in practice. Nor does it mean that the recipient never has the right to dispose of the object. The existence of the ability to recover a gift and of other possible rights and typical practices are empirical questions. What is important is that people think of the object as bearing the identity of the giver and of the relationship between the giver and the recipient.[34]

A failure to recognize this fact about freely given blood, organs, or other tissues is what leads to scandals like Alder Hey. It is not sufficient to keep market relations away from human goods if the rationalizing tendencies of formal organizations do just as good a job of taking distinct, particular, incommensurable gifts and processing them into general, homogeneous, comparable items.[35]

There are two moments of exchange in human goods. The tissues are first procured from donors or sellers. They are then passed to other organizations to be processed and distributed—according to some fixed system of distribution (as with solid organs), through a secondary market (as with some other tissues), or pursuant to some other set of rules. Very few human goods are nowadays passed directly from giver to recipient. A unit of blood is more likely than not to be fractionated and processed into many separate products that are more easily stored and more precisely targeted than whole blood. This processing tends to increase the distance between the giver and the gift, which comes to take on the quality of a generic item in the inventory of medical supplies. Outside of illegal markets or transnational trade in body parts, scandals involving human goods have generally arisen when primary gifts are thought to be defiled in secondary exchanges. Sometimes just the fact of this reprocessing is sufficient to make uninformed donors feel they have been betrayed.

The key interface is not the individual-to-individual transaction (largely a myth anyway) but the transition into the secondary exchange of human goods—the world where donated hearts go, where donated skin is rendered, and where knee joints and heart valves and tendons are processed. This organizational layer does not have the (even fictively) particularized quality that individual decisions to donate or sell may possess. It is concerned with maintaining a reliable supply of homogenous products to cope with demand. Though not inevitable, it should not be wholly surprising that a willed-body program would get into trouble for mixing donated bodies with medical waste and animal remains and dumping them in a landfill. That sort of tendency is built into complex organizations, and it persists whether or not the raw materials are obtained via markets or gifts. It is a consequence of the industrialization of exchange in human goods, not its commodification.

This means that, while we should worry about exploitation in the exchange of human goods, it is a mistake to think that commodification as such is the reason exploitation happens. Commodified exchanges may well be exploitative, but market exchange does not automatically make it so. Both gift and market systems depend on their specific institutional realization for their effects. The choice is not between morally worthwhile gift giving and morally evil markets. We can see this if we look at anthropological studies of illegal sales. The gray market for kidneys and corneas has properly been held up as a prime case of exploitation and abuse. But desperate organ sellers are not exploited simply because they contract a sale. Rather, it is the wider social context in which they find themselves—their dominated class position, long-term disadvantage, and poor life chances—that puts them in a situation that invites their exploitation by "transplant tourists." There is no contradiction in saying that people in such desperate circumstances may choose—and even be eager—to be exploited. In fact it is exactly in the cases where people's needs are greatest that they will be most prepared to voluntarily enter into a contract that exploits them. It is not the contract that is the source of the exploitation, however, but the willingness of the buyer to take advantage of another's vulnerability.[36] It is for the same reason, incidentally, that we are puzzled or even suspicious of relatively well off people who say they want to give a kidney to a stranger. When the need is much greater on the part of the potential recipient, the potential donor has nothing to gain materially from the transaction, and there is no social tie between them, then all of the vulnerability is on the recipient's side. Why then, we wonder, would the donor want to put herself at risk?

Systematic vulnerability on the donor side is of course much more common, and this is part of what makes a market in organs a worrying prospect. There are enough people who would consider selling one of their kidneys only because they are poor and desperate. There are two ways to prevent this kind of exploitation from happening. The first is to ban commercial exchange in human goods (and vigorously pursue violators), so that people will not have the opportunity to enter into exploitative contracts. The second is to redistribute bargaining power in such a way that any exchanges that do happen will not be exploitative. The problem with the first solution is that, as Allen Wood points out, it risks "consigning the vulnerable person to an even worse fate than being exploited."[37] The problem with the second solution is that it may be difficult to implement in practice, because it will generally involve questions of social justice that go well beyond any particular sale of blood or organs. Supporters of markets in human goods point to the first problem, arguing that nothing is gained by banning organ sales except a warm glow of moral satisfaction for those who will neither benefit nor suffer from such a ban. Opponents point to the second problem, arguing that in practice such markets would reinforce existing inequalities rather than ameliorating them.

The situation with cadaveric organs is, as always, more complex. The economic logic of organ sales is straightforward: there is a dollar price for organs at present—it is zero. If we forced people to *pay* to become organ donors, then we would expect the supply to drop. Therefore, there is no reason to believe that the supply would not rise if we gave families a small payment instead. But there are two complications, one arising from theory and one from empirical facts about procurement. The theoretical objection is that it is not clear the supply curve for cadaveric organs is linear around zero. Many people are prepared to carry out an action like organ donation for free, and there are perhaps also many people (maybe the same individuals) who would agree to a sale for a very large amount of money. But what if there are hardly any people who would agree to sell for a *small* amount of money? There is an analogy to bribery: We do not think that people who ask for modestly sized bribes are only a little bit more corrupt than people who do not ask for bribes at all. Instead, there is a sharp discontinuity. The intuition here is similar to the idea, discussed in chapter 1, that the market can "crowd out" voluntary action, that volunteers will leave the scene once financial incentives are introduced.[38] This objection, different but related, suggests that when the altruists are crowded out as suppliers, there may be no one available to take their place until prices are driven very high.

The empirical complication is that, at bottom, the supply of cadaveric donors is not responsive to financial incentives. People become potential donors when they die suddenly, in particular sorts of circumstances. None of the logistical problems discussed in chapter 3 go away when financial incentives are introduced. While payment might help lower the refusal rate, it cannot (absent some very perverse incentives) boost the raw supply. For cadaveric organs, all of the potential effect of market incentives is focused on those families who refuse consent. While money might make a difference at this stage, this is also the point where crowding out and similar effects are most likely to happen. And unlike other exchanges that have suffered from crowding out, there is no prospect of new suppliers moving into the market to replace those who leave.

For other kinds of human goods, avoiding exploitation means organizing the exchange in a way that prevents the recipient from being able to take advantage of weakness or vulnerability on the part of the supplier. Can the Maussian concept of the gift relationship offer any help with this problem? Rituals of gift giving can encourage people to think of exchange in blood and organs as establishing social ties between givers and recipients, despite the complex organizational intervention needed to make the transaction happen. To that extent, they link the demand for human goods to social relations more generally. They remind us that these goods are being exchanged between human beings, rather than coming from some abstract source that can simply be treated as a means to an end. As Titmuss argued, "Voluntary blood donor systems . . . represent one practical and concrete demonstration of fellowship relationships institutionally based in Britain in the National Health Service and the National Blood Transfusion Service."[39]

Yet just as a market relationship does not automatically make for exploitation, neither does a gift relationship automatically create solidarity. The structural relationships between suppliers, distributors, and recipients will affect how plausible the gift relationship is, in the same way that systematic social inequalities determine whether the pro forma equality of market transactions has any substantive basis. As we saw in chapter 5, the commercial plasma market globalized in the 1970s and 1980s in spite of a public commitment to voluntary donation on the part of blood collection agencies. Indeed, this very commitment was one of the forces behind that transformation. European blood collection agencies found that they could not find enough volunteer plasma donors to meet demand but were unwilling or unable to modify their gift-based systems. Instead, they began to purchase their plasma from commercial sources in the United States.[40] The subsequent AIDS disaster should remind us that social solidarity is not the goal of exchange in human goods: the system only exists in order that illness can be cured and lives saved. Solidarity is a by-product. It would be a bitter irony if a commitment to the gift relationship as public policy made people more rather than less likely to forget this fact.

When blood donation involved the transfer of whole blood from one person to another, and when the mediating organization was a National Health Service that aimed to serve everyone in the same way, then the sense of inclusion in society fostered by generalized exchange in blood was easier to feel. The whole circuit of exchange was visible to donors.

Things are now very different. There are many kinds of blood products and they have longer shelf lives. Collection organizations process their donations much more intensively, and secondary markets for the resulting products have proliferated. A parallel process is well under way for goods derived from cadaveric donors. These changes mean that supporters of gift-based exchange should be less worried about the prospect of reimbursing donors or donor families and more concerned with the effects of these rapidly expanding and highly profitable new markets. Particularly in the case of organ donation, donor families may be appalled to discover that the donation they have been strongly encouraged to think of as a unique, inalienable gift quickly became a commodity input to a production process. More broadly, inequalities in access to health care make it difficult to feel that there is a genuine process of generalized reciprocity at work, or some kind of broader social bargain that justifies donation.

Possible Futures

What is the future of exchange in human goods? There are many possibilities, of course: in fact, the variety of viable institutional arrangements is one of the lessons of this book. But assuming that demand for organs continues to rise and secondary markets for tissues continue to expand, we can think of four main paths that the exchange of human blood, organs, and tissues might take. The first is a shift to a purely market-driven system, where the raw materials are routinely sold for profit, with no pretence of gift exchange and none of the language of donation. The plasma market in the United States comes closest to this model and has operated in this fashion for many years. Instituting a similar arrangement for organ procurement would require revisiting and remaking the cultural account of donation. Because the account seems well entrenched, a smooth shift to a market system is unlikely. It is not out of the question, however; the life insurance market of the nineteenth century shows that profane financial considerations can be incorporated into the sacred world of death, and the growing pressure of demand might trigger a rapid reorientation of the system. But the distinctive circumstances of organ procurement make this more difficult to achieve than in other areas, even the blood market. The legalization of live organ suppliers (selling kidneys) is somewhat more likely, as in this case there are no family members to complicate the decision process.

The second option lies at the other end of the scale. This would involve a return to something as close as possible to the arrangement Titmuss described, where the gift exchange of blood and organs is relatively direct and, ideally, generates the kind of institutionally grounded social solidarity Titmuss argued for. In one sense this has happened already, as the U.S. blood supply moved away from paying suppliers of whole blood in the 1970s. Much like the child labor market in the nineteenth century, the decommodification of the U.S. blood market is a strong counterexample to the thesis that markets always and everywhere expand once they have taken hold. Yet as we saw, this reorganization happened just prior to a time of great technological change in the blood and tissue industries. The ensuing changes make it difficult to see how Titmuss's vision of the blood supply could return as a real, working arrangement. Blood and tissue markets are by now too large and too differentiated to be serviced solely by a version of Titmuss's ideal.

This suggests a third and more pessimistic alternative. The cultural account of donation may become increasingly entrenched, buttressed by the emphasis on individual autonomy and informed consent that animates the field of bioethics. In this way, a particular vision of purely voluntary donation would become the sine qua non for procurement. The presence of any kind of financial reimbursement would be taken as evidence that the donor's decision had been coerced or otherwise negatively influenced. The purity of the decision to give would thus be the cornerstone of the public legitimation of the system. Now, we are used to the close association of markets and individualism, and indeed critics of market society commonly point to its atomizing and alienating effects. But in the late nineteenth century Émile Durkheim observed the rise of the cult of the individual and argued that its origins lay not in the market as such, but in the division of labor more generally. He argued that, in modern societies, while "other beliefs and practices assume less and less religious a character, the individual becomes the object of a sort of religion." So while market incentives and altruistic motives are typically opposed to one another, from a different point of view they are two sides of the same collective commitment to the sovereignty of individual choice. The difficulty with this distinctively modern religion, Durkheim worried, is that "it is indeed from society that it draws all its strength, but it is not to society that it binds us: it is to ourselves."[41]

This outcome would combine a highly elaborated rhetoric of altruistic giving, on the procurement side, and a rapidly industrializing and profitable sector, on the distribution side. The emphasis on the wholly free gift would not mesh with the underlying social organization of the human goods industry. The Maussian elements of gift exchange, which emphasize the importance of gifts in terms of the social relations they express and sustain, would give way to the ideology of the pure gift, where what matters is that the gift is bestowed freely and with no strings attached. The result would be a kind of "gift fetishism" not all that different in substance from Marx's idea of commodity fetishism. Divorced from the true conditions of their production and distribution, pure gifts mask the social relations that link givers and recipients, and become imbued with powers they do not really have—such as the power to guarantee the fairness of an exchange or produce solidarity in a community.

In such circumstances, the world of human goods would become most saturated with a sacred reverence for the gift of human goods just at the moment scientific and technological development seemed set to reduce our image of the body to a soulless repository for spare parts. In this future, it would be technological developments themselves that made room for the sacralization of hearts, lungs, or livers. This tendency is already present in the cultural account of donation, and we see something like it at work in the world of stem-cell research and genetic engineering. There, the scientific capacity to isolate and grow small clumps of embryonic stem cells has opened the way for these entities to be invested (by some) with the same rights and protections granted to individuals. To the extent that a system of this sort emphasized the moment of individual choice rather than the subsequent social life of the gift, however, it would be vulnerable to the presence of chronic inequality in the health system as a whole. The ideology of the pure gift would be difficult to sustain in the long run, because the gap between the procurement system's rationale and its actual operation would allow public goodwill and support for donation to leach away. Given present trends, though, this may well be the most likely future for exchange in human goods.

A fourth possibility would see the introduction of money into the gift exchange of organs in some way, but without moving over to a system characterized only by financial incentives. The idea would be to provide some monetary compensation while retaining the giftlike features of the transaction. This is partly a way to emphasize the special nature of the transaction, and partly to allow for the development and expression of norms of fairness in exchange: if there is profit at every other point in the process, the giver ought to be compensated as well. The market for human eggs, for example, deals in among the most commercialized of human goods, and yet it is carried on using much of the language and form of gift exchange. An emphasis on donation, even when it is accompanied by payment, can be an assertion of a social relationship with particular rights and obligations on both sides. It is easy to be cynical about this and (as we saw in chapter 2) to assume that the gift elements are sheer facade or empty ritual. However, studies of egg donors suggest this is not the case. While the staff of donation agencies speak in openly economic terms about the quality of their donors (such as their attractiveness to buyers), they also emphasize that they are not brokering a simple commodity transaction. It is especially striking—and consistent with the growth of the cultural account of donation—that it is the agencies and not the donors who take the lead in emphasizing the giftlike elements in the exchange. Although the egg donors themselves often enter the process with only the payment in mind, the agency staff work to convince them that "they are not 'manufacturing toothpaste' or 'selling pens.' They also consistently refer to the women and men who produce genetic material as 'donors' who 'help' recipients by giving a very special 'gift.'"[42] While giftlike relationships of this kind are more likely to frame the exchange of human goods than other commodities, they are not limited to parts of the economy dealing in exotic or obviously sacred items. They can be found even where the interests of the contracting parties are essentially in conflict with one another. In labor markets, participants often strive to embed their contractual exchanges in institutions that insulate them from exploitation and perhaps also yield a higher return than straightforward competition.[43]

Regardless of which arrangement comes to pass—one of those laid out here, or some other arrangement—it is worth emphasizing again that broader questions about the distribution of power and resources between suppliers, recipients, and procurement organizations will play a decisive role in determining the quality of the outcome. Exploitation will not be avoided—and supply problems will not be solved—simply by making the exchange take one form or another.

———

In the next ten to twenty years, the scope of exchange in human goods goods will continue to expand. It is likely, though, that the supply of the most important raw material—cadaveric donors—will grow only slowly. Continuing technical advances in biotechnology and medical practice will put more and more pressure on the supply organizations to locate, procure, and process their products, absent a revolution in xenotransplantation or some other wholly novel technology.[44] Viewed historically, the long-term trend seems to be away from gift-based exchange, though the evidence that market incentives would outperform the current supply of cadaveric organs is weak. (Goods that can be supplied by live donors are a different matter.) Blood supply systems rely on volunteers for whole blood and its derivatives, but the plasma industry could not exist without paid suppliers. Organ procurement agencies face much more severe demand pressure from patients and doctors and have begun to experiment with financial incentives. Markets for sperm, eggs, and children are already thoroughly commercialized, though they are shot through with the language and forms of gift giving. It remains to be seen how exchange in cell derivatives and other genetic material will be organized, but there have already been a string of important decisions to secure private property rights in these goods—though not for the individuals who carry them.[45]

Gift-based systems of blood and organ donation provide a well-institutionalized model of exchange in human goods when individual donors or their families are directly involved. Although the performance of particular organizations varies, good organizational management of voluntary donors has the capacity to deliver close to the maximum possible number of donors. The development of this potential, however, has gone hand in hand with the expansion of profitable secondary markets in human goods. The cultural scripts and accounts that blood and organ suppliers draw on to legitimate their work also provide the chief resource for critiquing what happens to these gifts after they are collected. In a strong sense, procurement organizations produce the donor populations they rely on.

Titmuss argued that "the ways in which society organizes and structures its social institutions . . . can encourage or discourage the altruistic in man."[46] He thought that the introduction of market incentives drove out the disposition to be charitable, in a kind of Gresham's law of motives. Following his lead, Peter Singer suggests that we think of a quality like altruism as being a capacity or skill that becomes more available with regular use.[47] As this book has shown, this skill can be exercised in different ways and with varying results. Other human capacities have this quality of being able to improve and grow with use, particularly those clustering around concepts like civic-mindedness, benevolence, public-spiritedness, and love. "My bounty is as boundless as the sea," Juliet says to Romeo. "The more I give to thee, the more I have."[48] But we should not be overly optimistic about the power of these capacities. They presuppose a wider moral economy in which gifts and voluntary action are not routinely taken advantage of, and where the terms of individual exchanges are at least plausibly fair. The ongoing interaction between the social organization of the human goods industry and the cultural legitimacy of blood and organ donation is more complex than the continued cultivation of the capacity to give. Albert Hirschman describes it better when he observes that altruism and charity "exhibit a complex, composite behavior:

they atrophy when not adequately practiced and appealed to . . . yet will once again make themselves scarce when preached on and relied on to excess."[49] The aim of this book has not been to explain away the altruism of blood and organ donors by reducing it to some other psychological motive. Rather, I have argued that by analyzing the social basis of exchange in human goods, we can better understand how opportunities to give are successfully created by organizations in the short run. We can also learn how acts like this are culturally sustained and morally valued in the long run. The goal, in other words, has been to see which organizations make gifts best, and how institutions make gifts last.

Appendix: Data Sources and Methods

Chapter 2

I rely on three sources of data in this chapter. First, I examined promotional material, official reports, policy statements, and other discussion papers originating with organ procurement organizations or their coordinating agency, the United Network for Organ Sharing. Second, I collected a comprehensive sample of book-length journalistic accounts and personal memoirs of organ donation published between 1980 and 1999. These books began to appear with increasing frequency in the 1980s. The official sources reflect the interests of the OPOs in increasing the organ supply and represent their best efforts at convincing potential donors that giving organs is worthwhile. Like the early advocates of life insurance, the OPOs lay out arguments in favor of a practice that trespasses on questions of life and death in a disturbing way. The stories told in the popular books add narrative detail and emotional depth to these policy arguments. I argue that they act as a cultural resource, a way of familiarizing the public with the rules and ideals of this new practice. They publicize the experiences of those affected, providing rich, personalized narratives about donation to all involved. (References to these books can be found in the notes to the chapter.) Third, I sampled the *New York Times* (via the Lexis-Nexis database) for all stories appearing between January 1, 1980, and December 31, 1999, that had the words "organ" and "donor" or "transplant" in the headline or lead paragraph. The initial search yielded 1,012 news items for the twenty-year period. (After checking each story, 14 were eliminated as irrelevant. Most of these concerned the gift of a church organ in New York.) The median number of stories per year is 50, with a minimum of 9 (in 1980) and a maximum of 86 (in 1999). Figures 2.2 and 2.3 show smoothed estimates of percentage coverage in the *New York Times,* calculated using a running-median formula.

Chapter 3

The analysis of OPO procurement rates draws on a variety of data sources. Data on the absolute number of organs procured by each OPO each year are freely available. OPOs administer areas of widely differing sizes and populations, so this number needs to be standardized. As discussed in the chapter, there is some controversy about what the appropriate denominator is. The best available measure is *donors per thousand evaluable deaths.* The Centers for Disease Control and Prevention collect mortality statistics for the United States, and these statistics record causes of death. In a 1997 report on the organ transplant industry, the General Accounting Office listed those causes of death, defined by their ICD-9-CM mortality codes, that could be expected to yield a potential donor. (GAO, *Organ Procurement Organizations,* 1997). *Evaluable deaths* are the subset of all deaths in a given area whose ICD-9 code is one of those listed in the GAO report. The dependent variable in the analysis is the absolute number of donors procured by an OPO in 1997; procurement rate was determined by dividing that figure by the number of evaluable deaths and multiplying by a thousand. CDC mortality data are available at the county level. To calculate the number of evaluable deaths for each OPO, each observed county in the U.S. was given a code identifying its OPO. Then the number of evaluable deaths was summed for all counties with that code, thus aggregating observations for 3,142 counties to into figures for each of the 61 OPOs. The measures of population density (per square kilometer) and the percentage of those in regional populations who are black or poor or have college degrees are based on county-level reports by the U.S. Census Bureau, again aggregated to the OPO level. The original data are published in the Census Bureau's *U.S. County Data* 1998. Race and education figures were from 1996, poverty figures from 1993. County-level data on road deaths were extracted from the Federal Accident Reporting System and aggregated to OPO-level rates using population data from the Census Bureau.

Data on referring hospitals come from appendix V of GAO, *Organ Transplants* (1993). These figures are for 1991–92. Some OPOs changed their names or merged with others between then and 1997. Information from UNOS was used to reconcile the two lists. Data on the spending and staff structures of OPOs were compiled from Medicare cost-reimbursement reports submitted to the Health Care Financing Authority (now known as the Centers for Medicare and Medicaid Services) for 1997. Spending was calculated from the Total Administrative Expenses worksheet of these reports. In the models, spending is denominated in hundreds of dollars per capita. Case-by-case data on the procurement policies of OPOs in the United States come from a telephone survey of OPOs conducted in 1999. The original analysis of some of the questions can be found in Wendler and Dickert, "Consent Process for Cadaveric Organ Procurement" (2001). The authors kindly supplied me with their final data file for the survey and the text of the survey instrument.

Although I do not try to estimate their effects, three other features of the OPO's environment should be mentioned. The first is state law. States have implemented several kinds of laws that may affect organ procurement rates. Soon after the passing of the National Organ Transplantation Act in 1984, states begin to provide organ donor cards on the back of drivers licenses. In the late 1980s, most states also enacted "required request" laws, which require hospitals to consult with a potential donor's next of kin should the patient be near death. These laws are generally agreed not to have increased donation rates (Norris, "Required Request," 1990). A number of studies have shown that, about a quarter of the time, eligible families are not offered the option to donate (Gortmaker, "Organ Donor Potential," 1996). Several states have passed "routine notification" laws, which require that all deaths, actual or imminent, be referred to the local OPO. There is evidence that this has increased procurement rates in some areas (H. M. Nathan, "Pennsylvania Looks for Answers to the Organ Donor Shortage," Gift of Life Program press release, Pittsburgh, 1999; T. J. Shafer, "Two Years Experience with Routine Notification," paper presented at the annual meeting of the North American Transplant Coordinators Organization, New York, August 10, 1998). Because over-time data are not available for some of the important variables, I do not try to estimate the effects of these laws here.

Second, religious participation and affiliation may affect one's likelihood of supporting donation, or of consenting given the opportunity. Existing research on religion has focused on the theological or traditional objections some religions have or have had to organ donation (Abraham Twersky, Michael Gold, and Walter Jacob, "Jewish Perspectives," and David Kelly and Walter Wiest, "Christian Perspectives," both in C. Don Keyes and Walter E. Wiest, eds. *New Harvest: Transplanting the Body and*

Reaping the Benefits [Clifton: Humana Press, 1991]). There has been no research on whether the geography of religious affiliation maps onto variation in donation rates. The literature on religious attitudes toward organ donation might suggest that areas with large numbers of Jews, Conservative Catholics, and members of some Protestant denominations would have lower donation rates. I used county-level data on religious affiliation and activity to examine whether there was a link between religion and procurement. The data came from M. B. Bradley et al., "Churches and Church Membership in the United States" (Washington, DC: Glenmary Research Center, 1992). Exploratory analyses did not show any strong effects, however.

Third, the geographical distribution of OPO procurement rates is quite suggestive. As can be seen from figure 3.4 in the main text, OPOs in the upper Midwest do especially well. It is possible that organ donation lines up with other measures of associational activity and social capital more broadly (Robert Putnam, *Bowling Alone: The Collapse and Revival of American Community* [New York: Simon and Schuster, 2000]). It would be rash to generalize too confidently, however, given the complex organizational basis of donor procurement and the limits of the available data. While exploratory analysis did not indicate either a statistically significant degree of spatial clustering in the data or a strong relationship to the density of voluntary organizations within OPO catchment areas, further study of the geography of organ procurement is certainly needed.

The models in columns 1 and 2 of table A.1 employ a robust MM-estimator and were generated using the rlm function in R (W. N. Venables and B. D. Ripley, *Modern Applied Statistics with S,* 4th ed. [New York: Springer, 2002], 161–63; R Core Development Team, "R: A Language and Environment for Statistical Computing" [Vienna: R Foundation for Statistical Computing, 2003]). Model 1 predicts procurement rates in 1997 using variables that measure features of the OPOs' catchment areas. Model 2 adds organizational-level measures. Estimating the robust model gives a valid N of 44 rather than 61, due to missing data. Given that the deleted cases are missing data on only one or two variables, and the number of observations is small, it is preferable to make use of all of the available data. I used multiple imputation to predict values for the missing data. The algorithm applied here uses additive regression and predictive mean matching to impute values for missing data. Variance and covariance estimates are weighted to account for the fact that the model is estimated from partly imputed data. The multiple imputation and model estimation procedures are described in more detail in Frank E. Harrell, *Regression Modeling Strategies* (New York: Springer, 2001; pp. 47–50, 69–70) and implemented in his

TABLE A.1. **Models predicting donor procurement rates**

Variable	(1)	(2)	(3)
(Intercept)	52.907	3.109	1.331
	(5.10)	(0.19)	(0.08)
Pop. density (log)	5.174	6.574	6.319
	(3.14)	(4.27)	(4.39)
Percent black	−0.325	−0.298	−0.333
	(−2.24)	(−2.20)	(−2.57)
Percent poor	−0.937	−0.616	−0.582
	(−2.53)	(−1.65)	(−1.77)
Percent college	−1.134	−0.957	−0.840
	(−2.51)	(−2.30)	(−2.12)
OPO spending (log)		9.359	9.243
		(3.04)	(2.96)
Referrers		0.149	0.183
		(2.31)	(2.88)
OPO policy		−0.040	−0.011
		(−0.20)	(−0.05)
Adjusted R^2	0.336	0.534	0.443
Valid N	61	44	61

Notes: Models (1) and (2) employ a resistant MM-estimator. Model (3) employs multiple imputation. *T*-values are in parentheses below coefficients.

Hmisc library for R, which was used to generate the model reported in column 3 of the table. Figure 3.4 shows predicted effects derived from model 3 in table A.1 and was produced using functions from the Hmisc library.

Chapter 4

The data analysis in this chapter is based on data on blood donation across Europe from a survey carried out in Europe in 1994 (Reif and Marlier, *Eurobarometer 41.0,* 1995). The survey sampled persons aged fifteen years and over residing in the twelve member states of the European Union, as well as Norway and Finland, and included thirty-one questions about blood donation and related issues. Respondents were asked for their opinions about the way blood and plasma are collected and handled, their reasons for donating and not donating, their understanding of the differences between blood and plasma, and their attitudes about buying and selling blood. The survey was carried out through multistage national probability samples and national stratified quota samples during March through June 1994. The complete dataset contains 19,477 cases. Finland is not included in this analysis because all blood-related data for this country were missing.

TABLE A.2. **Individual-level variables predicting blood donation**

Variable	Description
Female	Coded 1 for Female, 0 for Male.
Age	Age in Years. Centered on 35-year-olds.
Education	Years of full-time education. Centered on respondents with 16 years of full-time education.
Income	Eurobarometer's comparative income variable, ranging from 1 (lowest) to 12 (highest). This variable harmonizes income scores measured in different currencies.
Ties	A four-category code measuring contacts with transfusion recipients (including oneself). Values range from 0 (no ties) to 3 (ties to self, relative and friend).
Student	Coded 1 if the respondent is a student.

The individual-level variables are described in table A.2. Variables were coded with reference to the "modal donor" reported in research on donors discussed in the text. The Ties variable is constructed from a series of questions that asked respondents whether they themselves had ever received a blood transfusion, or whether they knew of a family member or a friend who had ever gotten one. The variables have been centered in order to give a substantive interpretation to the intercept term in the models. Age has been centered on thirty-five-year-olds and education on those with six-teen years of full-time education. Income has been centered on the top quartile threshold. The intercept therefore represents a thirty-five-year-old male in the top income quartile, with (roughly) a college education, who is currently not a student, and who has no network ties to transfusion recipients.

Table A.3 reports country-by-country results for a model where the dependent variable is whether the respondent has ever given blood. Other models, not reported here, tested the relationship between characteristics such as regular church attendance and membership in a union, and the probability of having donated blood in the past year. In general, these variables were significant predictors of recent donation.

Next, the institutional setting is represented by three variables. The first is the kind of collection system a country operates, as enumerated in the chapter. Countries with state-run systems make up the omitted category. The second is a binary variable registering the presence of a volunteer donor group in a country. Individuals from countries with such groups (Denmark, France, Greece, Italy, and Spain) are coded 1, others get a 0. In table A.4, the mixed-effects model specifies a country-level random effect to account for the fact that observations from the same country are not properly independent of one another. Substantively, the random effect accounts for unmeasured factors associated with each country, thereby providing a more conservative estimate than in the usual regression

TABLE A.3. **Country-level models of donation**

Country	Intercept	Female	Age	Education	Income	Ties	Student	N
State systems								
Britain	−0.299	−0.376	0.007	0.037	0.03	0.037	−0.694	694
	(−1.64)	(−2.27)	(1.37)	(1.29)	(1.15)	(0.3)	(−1.39)	
France	0.559	−0.712	0.004	0.125	0.077	0.336	−0.95	829
	(3.53)	(−4.73)	(0.74)	(5.11)	(3.27)	(3.25)	(−3.36)	
Ireland	0.092	−0.421	0.009	0.126	0.148	0.171	−1.771	542
	(0.35)	(−2.08)	(1.23)	(2.53)	(3.98)	(1.09)	(−2.27)	
Red Cross systems								
Belgium	−1.52	−0.583	0.007	0.043	−0.022	0.401	0.065	528
	(−5.94)	(−2.57)	(1.12)	(2.1)	(−0.58)	(2.56)	(0.15)	
Luxembourg	−1.359	−0.681	0	0.004	0.075	0.108	−1.686	378
	(−4.91)	(−2.2)	(0.04)	(0.1)	(1.62)	(0.58)	(−1.57)	
Netherlands	−0.715	−0.789	0.006	0.005	0.022	0.287	−0.416	856
	(−4.85)	(−4.91)	(1.16)	(0.27)	(0.96)	(2.48)	(−1.23)	
Germany	−0.622	−0.619	−0.007	0.047	0.045	0.529	−0.639	1707
	(−5.86)	(−5.6)	(−1.97)	(3.74)	(2.54)	(6.61)	(−2.22)	
Blood banking systems								
Denmark	−0.426	−0.584	0.013	0.047	0.047	0.161	−0.619	898
	(−3.09)	(−3.97)	(2.65)	(3.14)	(2.11)	(1.52)	(−2.04)	
Norway	−1.326	−0.329	0.012	0.032	0.167	0.365	−0.857	856
	(−7.37)	(−1.69)	(1.74)	(2.51)	(5.04)	(2.93)	(−1.82)	
Italy	−0.778	−1.09	0.003	0.04	0.004	0.279	−0.866	707
	(−3.62)	(−5.49)	(0.4)	(1.8)	(0.1)	(1.8)	(−2.29)	
Greece	0.914	−1.925	−0.018	0.021	0.086	0.325	−2.095	763
	(4.47)	(−10.61)	(−3.04)	(0.98)	(2.49)	(2.32)	(−5.64)	
Spain	−0.757	−0.553	0.003	0.036	0.038	0.214	−1.231	679
	(−3.81)	(−2.94)	(0.51)	(1.51)	(1.23)	(1.44)	(−2.82)	
Portugal	−1.06	−1.653	0.01	0.025	0.079	0.435	−2.081	805
	(−4.27)	(−7.27)	(1.43)	(1.02)	(2.13)	(2.39)	(−2.74)	

Note: T-statistics are given in parentheses below coefficients.

model of the institutional-level variables, which vary across countries. The interaction effects can be interpreted as showing how different institutional mechanisms modify the effect of individual characteristics on donation. The dependent variable in this model is whether the respondent has ever given blood. The model was fitted using the glmmPQL function in R (R Core Development Team, "R," 2003).

Chapter 5

The data for this chapter come mainly from an archive held at the library of the National Research Council in Washington, DC. In the wake of the

TABLE A.4. **Mixed-effects model of donation**

| | | Interaction Effects | | |
| | Main effect | Red Cross | Blood banks | Donor groups |
Variables				
Intercept	−0.240			
	(−1.14)			
Female	−0.436	−0.220	−0.431	−0.183
	(−4.10)	(−1.65)	(−3.42)	(−1.46)
Age	0.008	−0.009	0.000	−0.007
	(2.26)	(−2.09)	(0.06)	(−1.83)
Education	0.071	−0.045	−0.045	0.018
	(3.95)	(−2.46)	(−2.46)	(1.32)
Income	0.090	−0.05	−0.007	0.035
	(5.13)	(−2.41)	(−0.37)	(−1.72)
Ties	0.161	0.242	0.092	0.035
	(2.05)	(2.49)	(1.02)	(0.43)
Student	−0.957	0.765	−0.069	0.231
	(−2.99)	(2.05)	(−0.23)	(0.72)
Red Cross	−0.827			
	(−3.53)			
Blood bank	−0.431			
	(−3.42)			
Donor group	0.828			
	(3.53)			

Notes: Valid $N = 10{,}394$. Model is for population aged 18 and over. State system is the omitted category. T–statistics are given in parentheses below coefficients.

HIV disaster, activists and critics of the blood and plasma industry campaigned for a full Senate investigation of the matter. Instead, in 1994 the government directed the Institute of Medicine to investigate. The investigating committee held some public hearings and invited interested parties to submit arguments and information. However, all its interviews with blood industry executives were conducted in private. In addition to interviews, it obtained access to internal memos, the minutes or transcripts of meetings, and other previously confidential documents. The committee published its report in 1995.

The archive at the NRC contains copies of all of the documents received by the committee, as well as the notes made during face-to-face or telephone interviews with the principal players. These notes are not transcripts, though they often contain verbatim statements from interviewees along with summaries, paraphrases, and observations by the interviewer. Other than in the committee's own report, these data have not been analyzed before now. It is the best available window into the events of the period. If a relevant quotation appears in the Institute of Medicine report,

I cite it from there rather than the original documents, for convenience. Otherwise, I provide a direct reference to the archives.

The bulk of the information in the NRC archives concerns the internal workings of the Red Cross, blood banks, plasma companies, and the National Hemophilia Foundation. I also draw on the official transcript of the public hearings held by the committee in September 1994. This meeting heard evidence from victims of the disaster, mainly hemophiliacs and their families. See Committee to Study HIV Transmission through Blood Products, "Proceedings of a Public Meeting Held on September 12, 1994, in Washington D.C. (Department of Commerce, 1994).

Notes

CHAPTER ONE

1. For a survey of trends in the commodification of human bod-
    ies see the essays in Nancy Scheper-Hughes and Loïc Waquant,
    eds., *Commodifying Bodies* (Thousand Oaks, CA: Sage, 2002).
    Reports and analysis of the global trade in human organs can
    be found in Nancy Scheper-Hughes, "The Global Traffic in
    Human Organs," *Current Anthropology* 41, no. 2 (2000): 191–
    211, and Lawrence Cohen, "Where It Hurts: Indian Material
    for an Ethics of Organ Transplantation," *Dædalus* 128, no. 4
    (1999): 135–66.
2. Lori Andrews and Dorothy Nelkin, *Body Bazaar: The Market for
    Human Tissue in the Biotechnology Age* (New York: Crown,
    2001).
3. Douglas Starr, *Blood: An Epic History of Medicine and Commerce*
    (New York: Knopf, 1998).
4. P. Schmidt, "Blood and Disaster: Supply and Demand," *New
    England Journal of Medicine* 346 (2002): 617–20.
5. Stuart Bauer, "Blood Farming," *New York,* May 19, 1975, 50–70;
    Phillip Caputo, "Blood Banks: Pay Stations," *Chicago Tribune,*
    September 14, 1971; L. K. Altman, "Use of Commercial Blood
    Increases with Shortages in U.S.," *New York Times,* September 5,
    1970, A1, A12.
6. Starr, *Blood,* 231–49.
7. Ruth Richardson, "Fearful Symmetry: Corpses for Anatomy,
    Organs for Transplant?," in Stuart J. Younger, Renée C. Fox,
    and Laurence J. O'Connell, eds., *Organ Transplantation: Mean-
    ings and Realities* (Madison: University of Wisconsin Press,
    1996), 66–100.
8. Andrew Kimbrell, *The Human Body Shop: The Cloning, Engineer-*

ing and Marketing of Life, 2nd ed. (Washington, DC: Regnery, 1998). Jeremy Rifkin, *The Biotech Century* (New York: Tarcher, 1999).

9. Nancy Scheper-Hughes, *Parts Unknown: The Global Traffic in Human Organs* (New York: Farrar, Strauss and Giroux, forthcoming).

10. Karl Marx, *Capital* (London: Penguin, 1990), 1:758–872.

11. "The mysterious character of the commodity-form consists . . . in the fact that the commodity reflects the social characteristics of men's own labour as objective characteristics of the products of labour themselves. . . . [T]he definite social relation between men themselves . . . assumes here, for them, the fantastic form of a relation between things." Marx, *Capital,* 1:164–65.

12. G. A. Cohen, *Karl Marx's Theory of History: A Defence,* expanded ed. (Princeton: Princeton University Press, 2000), 115–33.

13. Marx, *Capital,* 1:179.

14. Marx, *Capital,* 1:367.

15. Karl Marx, "Inaugural Address of the International Working Men's Association," in *The Marx-Engels Reader,* 2nd ed., ed Robert C. Tucker, 517 (New York: Norton, 1978).

16. Karl Marx, "Wage-Labour and Capital," in *Karl Marx: Selected Writings,* ed. David McLellan, 275 (London: Oxford University Press, 2000).

17. Karl Marx, "On James Mill," in McLellan, *Karl Marx,* 124.

18. Marx, *Capital,* 1:920, 926.

19. Arguments about the problem of commodification are thriving in many fields, including philosophy, law, economics, sociology, anthropology, and public health. Notable contributions include Elizabeth Anderson, *Value in Ethics and Economics* (Cambridge, MA: Harvard University Press, 1993); Margaret Radin, *Contested Commodities* (Cambridge, MA: Harvard University Press, 1996); Martha Nussbaum, "'Whether from Reason or Prejudice': Taking Money for Bodily Services," *Journal of Legal Studies* 27 (June 1998): 693–724; Cass Sunstein, *Free Markets and Social Justice* (New York: Oxford University Press, 1997); Julie Nelson, "One Sphere or Two?," *American Behavioral Scientist* 41, no. 10 (1998): 1467–71; Peter Ubel, *Pricing Life* (Cambridge, MA: MIT Press, 2000); and Scheper-Hughes and Waquant, *Commodifying Bodies.* This work continues (not always directly) an earlier wave of debate that began in the 1970s. See especially Richard Titmuss, *The Gift Relationship: From Human Blood to Social Policy* (New York: Vintage, 1971); Kenneth Arrow, "Gifts and Exchanges," *Philosophy and Public Affairs* 1, no. 4 (1972): 343–62; Peter Singer, "Altruism and Commerce: A Defense of Titmuss Against Arrow," *Philosophy and Public Affairs* 2, no. 3 (1973): 312–20; Elizabeth Landes and Richard Posner, "The Economics of the Baby Shortage," *Journal of Legal Studies* 7 (1978): 323–48; and Michael Walzer, *Spheres of Justice* (New York: Basic Books, 1983). The goal throughout has been to determine exactly what commodification is, what it does to people and goods, and which things—if any—should be kept from the market.

20. The classic statement of this last idea is Karl Polanyi, *The Great Transformation: The Political and Economic Origins of Our Time* (Boston: Beacon Press, 1980).

21. Radin, *Contested Commodities;* Anderson, *Value in Ethics and Economics.*

22. Jon Elster, "Selfishness and Altruism," in *Beyond Self-Interest,* edited by Jane J. Mansbridge (Chicago: University of Chicago Press, 1990), 44-53.

23. Arjun Appadurai, "Commodities and the Politics of Value," in *The Social Life of Things,* ed. Arjun Appadurai, 26 (Cambridge: Cambridge University Press, 1986).

24. Walzer, *Spheres of Justice,* 100.

25. Viviana Zelizer, "The Purchase of Intimacy," *Law and Social Inquiry* 25, no. 3 (2000): 817-48. For further analysis of the role of the market in caring relationships, see, for example, Reva B. Siegel, "The Modernization of Marital Status Law: Adjudicating Wives' Rights to Earnings, 1860-1930," *Georgetown Law Journal* 82 (September 1994): 2127-2211; Katharine Silbaugh, "Turning Labor into Love: Housework and the Law," *Northwestern University Law Review* 91 (1996): 1-85; and Joan Williams, *Unbending Gender: Why Family and Work Conflict and What To Do about It* (New York: Oxford University Press, 1999).

26. Arlie Russell Hochschild, *The Commercialization of Intimate Life* (Berkeley: University of California Press, 2003).

27. Jon Elster, *Sour Grapes* (New York: Cambridge University Press, 1983), 1-42.

28. See, for example Charles E. Lindblom, *The Market System* (New Haven: Yale University Press, 2002) pp. 1-52.

29. Daniel M. Hausman and Michael S. McPherson, *Economic Analysis and Moral Philosophy* (New York: Cambridge University Press, 1996).

30. Roger Blair and David Kaserman, "The Economics and Ethics of Alternative Cadaveric Organ Procurement Policies," *Yale Journal of Regulation* 8 (1991): 403-52; Henry Hansmann, "The Economics and Ethics of Markets for Human Organs," *Journal of Health Politics, Policy and Law* 14 (1989): 57-85.

31. Richard Titmuss, *The Gift Relationship: From Human Blood to Social Policy,* expanded and updated ed. (New York: New Press, 1997).

32. B. S. Frey, F. OberholzerGee and R. Eichenberger, "The Old Lady Visits Your Backyard: A Tale of Morals and Markets," *Journal of Political Economy* 104, no. 6 (1996): 1297-1313; Bruno Frey, "A Constitution for Knaves Crowds out Civic Virtues," *Economic Journal* 107 (1997): 1043-53.

33. "The amount offered varied between SFr 2,500 per individual and year (N = 117), to SFr 5,000 (N = 102), and SFr 7,500 (N = 86) which is substantial in view of a median household income of our respondents of SFr 63,000 per year." Frey, "Constitution for Knaves," 1047.

34. Walzer, *Spheres of Justice.*

35. Radin, *Contested Commodities,* 114.

36. Radin, *Contested Commodities,* 122.

37. Gerald Marwell and Ruth Ames, "Economists Free Ride: Does Anyone Else?" *Journal of Public Economics* 15 (1981): 295-310; Robert Frank, Thomas Gilovich, and Dennis Regan, "Does Studying Economics Inhibit Cooperation?" *Journal of Economic Perspectives* 7 (1993): 159-72.

38. Viviana Zelizer, *The Social Meaning of Money* (New York: Basic Books, 1994).

39. Zelizer, *Social Meaning of Money,* 17 (emphasis in original).

40. Robert Wuthnow, *Acts of Compassion: Caring for Others and Helping Ourselves* (Princeton: Princeton University Press, 1991), *Learning to Care: Elementary Kindness in an Age of Indifference* (New York: Oxford University Press, 1995), and *Poor Richard's Principle: Recovering the American Dream through the Moral Dimension of Work, Business, and Money* (Princeton: Princeton University Press, 1996).

41. Wuthnow, *Acts of Compassion,* 84–88.

42. Dale Miller, "The Norm of Self Interest," *American Psychologist* 54, no. 12 (1999): 1–8; Dale T. Miller and Rebecca Ratner, "The Power of the Myth of Self-Interest," in *Current Societal Issues In Justice,* ed. L. Montada and M. Lerner, 25–48 (New York: Plenum Press, 1996).

43. Stephanie Strom, "An Organ Donor's Generosity Raises the Question of How Much Is Too Much?" *New York Times,* August 17, 2003, A14; Stephanie Strom, "Extreme Philanthropy: Giving of Yourself, Literally, to People You've Never Met," *New York Times,* July 27, 2003, D3.

44. Lichang Lee, Jane Allyn Piliavin, and Vaughn R. A. Call, "Giving Time, Money and Blood: Similarities and Differences," *Social Psychology Quarterly* 62 (1999): 276–90; Jane Allyn Piliavin and Peter L. Callero, *Giving Blood: The Development of an Altruistic Identity* (Baltimore: Johns Hopkins University Press, 1991).

45. Marcel Mauss, *The Gift: The Form and Reason for Exchange in Archaic Societies* (New York: Norton, 2000); Bronislaw Malinowski, *Crime and Custom in Savage Society* (London: Routledge, 1926); Bronislaw Malinowski, *Argonauts of the Western Pacific* (London: Routledge, 1922).

46. Peter Ekeh, *Social Exchange Theory: The Two Traditions* (Cambridge, MA: Harvard University Press, 1974); Marhsall Sahlins, *Stone Age Economics* (Chicago: Aldine, 1972); C. A. Gregory, *Gifts and Commodities* (London: Academic Press, 1982); Jonathan Parry and Maurice Bloch, eds., *Money and the Morality of Exchange* (Cambridge: Cambridge University Press, 1989); Annette Weiner, *Inalienable Possessions: The Paradox of Keeping-while-Giving* (Berkeley: University of California Press, 1992); Maurice Godelier, *The Enigma of the Gift* (Chicago: University of Chicago Press, 1999).

47. James Carrier, "Gifts, Commodities and Social Relations: A Maussian View of Exchange," *Sociological Forum* 6 (1991): 122.

48. Carrier, "Gifts, Commodities and Social Relations," 19–37; C. A. Gregory, "Gifts to Men and Gifts to God: Gift Exchange and Capital Accumulation in Contemporary Papua," *Man* 15 (1980): 626–52.

49. Malinowski, *Crime and Custom,* 42. See also Malinowski, *Argonauts.*

50. Mauss, *Gift,* 65.

51. Carrier, "Gifts, Commodities and Social Relations," 125.

52. Mauss, *Gift,* 66.

53. In Godelier's words: "*Why* is the debt created by a gift not cancelled or erased by an identical counter-gift? The answer . . . is basically simple. If the counter-gift does not erase the debt, it is because the 'thing' given has not

really been separated, completely detached, from the giver. The thing has been *given* without really being 'alienated' by the giver. The thing given therefore takes with it something of the person, of the identity of the giver. . . . The debt creates an obligation to give in return, but to give in return does not mean to give back, to repay; it means to give in turn. . . . Gift-giving in these societies is not simply a mechanism for setting possessions and people in circulation. . . . It is also, on a deeper level, the condition for the production and reproduction of the social relations . . . which characterize the bonds that are formed between individuals and groups" (Godelier, *Enigma of the Gift,* 42; emphasis in original). See also Weiner, *Inalienable Possessions.*

54. Mauss, *Gift,* 3.
55. John H. Evans, *Playing God? Human Genetic Engineering and the Rationalization of Bioethics, 1959-1995* (Chicago: University of Chicago Press, 2001); Onora O'Neill, *Autonomy and Trust in Bioethics* (Cambridge: Cambridge University Press, 2002).
56. Wendy Nelson Espeland and Mitchell L. Stevens, "Commensuration as a Social Process," *Annual Review of Sociology* 24 (1998): 315.
57. Cass Sunstein, "Incommensurability and Kinds of Valuation," in *Incommensurability, Incomparability and Practical Reason,* ed. Ruth Chang (Cambridge, MA: Harvard University Press, 1997), 238. Strictly speaking, there is more than this to the idea. *Incommensurable* items do not share a common scale of value along which they can be compared. One might think that if two goods are incommensurable they would also be *incomparable,* but this is not so. Item A can be better than item B without being *x* number of units better. Incommensurable goods can still be ordinally ranked, even if they cannot be cardinally valued. Incomparability is therefore a stronger idea than incommensurability. See the essays in Chang, *Incommensurability, Incomparability and Practical Reason,* for the nuances uncovered by philosophers working on this topic.
58. Michel Callon, ed., *The Laws of the Market* (Oxford: Blackwell, 1998); Bruce Carruthers and Arthur Stinchcombe, "The Social Structure of Liquidity: Flexibility, Markets and States," *Theory and Society* 28 (1999): 353-82.
59. Kristen Renwick Monroe, *The Heart of Altruism* (Princeton: Princeton University Press, 1998); S. P. Oliner and P. M. Oliner, *The Altruistic Personality: Rescuers of Jews in Nazi Europe* (New York: Free Press, 1988).

CHAPTER TWO

1. Wuthnow, *Poor Richard's Principle;* Marvin B. Scott and Stanford M. Lyman, "Accounts," *American Sociological Review* 33, no. 1 (1968): 46-62.
2. Arlie Hochschild, *The Managed Heart: Commercialization of Human Feeling* (Berkeley: University of California Press, 1985).
3. Viviana Zelizer, "Human Values and the Market: The Case of Life-Insurance and Death in 19th Century America," *American Journal of Sociology* 84 (1978):

591–610, and *Morals and Markets: The Development of Life Insurance in the United States* (New York: Columbia University Press, 1979).

4. The true size of the waiting list can be overstated. It is possible for a patient to register at more than one transplant center in the hope of increasing their chances of a transplant. Thus the number of registrations is higher than the number of candidates. The figure cited here refers to the number of candidates for transplantation—that is, to distinct individual patients.

5. Living donors make up an important and increasing proportion of donors, especially for kidney transplants and more recently (though in much smaller numbers) for liver transplants. Of course there can be no living donors when, as with hearts, people do not have one to spare.

6. Renée Fox and Judith Swazey, *The Courage to Fail: A Social View of Organ Transplantation and Dialysis* (Chicago: University of Chicago Press, 1974); Roberta Simmons, Susan Klein Marine, and Richard Simmons, *Gift of Life: The Social and Psychological Impact of Organ Transplantation* (New York: Wiley, 1977); Renée Fox and Judith Swazey, *Spare Parts: Organ Replacement in American Society* (New York: Oxford University Press, 1992).

7. On money management in personal relations see Nelson, "One Sphere or Two?"

8. Zelizer, *Morals and Markets.*

9. Zelizer, "Human Values and the Market," 598.

10. Zelizer, *The Social Meaning of Money,* 292.

11. Zelizer, "Human Values and the Market," 598, 605.

12. Richardson, "Fearful Symmetry," 68. Richardson goes on to describe how, in the eighteenth and nineteenth centuries, "those who procured corpses for dissection were known as 'resurrectionists' or 'bodysnatchers.' They operated largely on a black market and were reviled by the public. Dissection was viewed as a fate worse than death. In England, its negative associations were exacerbated by the fact that the bodies of condemned criminals were legally available for dissection. The poor were also especially at risk, as the bodies of those who died in workhouses or could not pay their funeral expenses became the property of the state, and were used for medical purposes."

13. Margaret Lock, "Deadly Disputes: Ideologies and Brain Death in Japan," in *Organ Transplantation: Meanings and Realities,* ed. Stuart J. Younger, Reneé Fox, and Laurence J. O'Connell, 142–67 (Madison: University of Wisconsin Press, 1996).

14. Linda Hogle, *Recovering the Nation's Body: Cultural Memory, Medicine and the Politics of Redemption* (New Brunswick, NJ: Rutgers University Press, 1999); Margaret Lock, *Twice Dead: Organ Transplants and the Reinvention of Death* (Berkeley: University of California Press, 2002).

15. In discussing the material put out by OPOs, I do not mean to suggest that there is no debate among transplant professionals regarding the best procurement strategies. There have in fact been three contending proposals: (1) to increase the donor pool by more aggressively pursuing "non-heart-beating"

donors (potential donors who are brain dead but not on life-support machines), (2) to eliminate refusals by curtailing the rights of donors or (especially) their families to veto harvesting, and (3) to introduce some monetary reward. Proposals of the first type are gaining support in the profession but threaten to undermine years of effort to educate the public about brain death. Those in the second category tend not to have much support. I deal with proposals of the third type below. I also show that, at different times, there has been some uncertainty amongst OPOs about which altruistic strategies would work best. See the appendix for details on the data used in this chapter.

16. Quoted in Zelizer, *Morals and Markets,* 294.

17. United Network for Organ Sharing, "Share Your Life. Share Your Decision," informational brochure (1999).

18. For example, motor vehicle accidents caused the death of 26 percent of cadaveric donors in 1997. Homicide or suicide victims accounted for a further 15 percent.

19. John Pekkanen, *Donor: how one girl's death gave life to others* (Boston: Little, Brown, 1986); Mary Zimmeth Schomaker, *Lifeline: How One Night Changed Five Lives* (New York: New Horizon Press, 1995); Reg Green, *The Nicholas Effect: A Boy's Gift to the World* (Sebastopol, CA: O'Reilly, 1999). See also Lee Gutkind, *Many Sleepless Nights: The World of Organ Transplantation* (Pittsburgh: University of Pittsburgh Press, 1990). Other books, with varying perspectives, include Phillip Dossick, *Transplant: A Family Chronicle* (New York: Viking, 1978); Elizabeth Parr, *I'm Glad You're Not Dead: A Liver Transplant Story* (New York: Journey, 1996); Thomas Starzl, *The Puzzle People: Memoirs of a Transplant Surgeon* (Pittsburgh: University of Pittsburgh Press, 1992); Nicholas Royle, *The Matter of the Heart* (London: Abacus, 1997); and Parichehr Yomtoob and Ted Schwarz, *The Gift of Life* (New York: St. Martin's Press, 1986).

20. Exactly how many requests are refused is difficult to measure. See Steven L. Gortmaker, "Improving the Request Process to Increase Family Consent for Organ Donation," *Journal of Transplant Coordination* 8 (1998): 210–17. I address the question of procurement methods in the next chapter.

21. The Transweb Memorial (http://www.transweb.org/) has memorials and comments from the next of kin of many donors.

22. Mauss, *Gift.* See also Godelier, *Enigma of the Gift,* 12.

23. We should remember, however, that those who decide to donate organs almost always do so because some sudden, violent event has caused the death of their next of kin. Why should Green's decision appear more noble to us than a similar decision made by a Los Angeles father whose son's organs are distributed to recipients in New York? The donors and recipients stand in the same relationship to one another in both cases (accidental victims, blameless recipients). The fact the event happened in a foreign country makes a larger difference to our moral judgments than perhaps it ought to. But it is precisely

these considerations—closeness of tie, link to a community, membership in a group—that we use to guide our evaluations of generosity and altruism.

24. From the Transweb memorial for Carl Zimmerman.

25. Hochschild, *Managed Heart.*

26. Karen Carney, *Precious Gifts: Katie Coolican's Story. Barklay and Eve Explain Organ and Tissue Donation* (n.p.: Dragonfly Publishing, 1999); Lizzy Ribal, *Lizzy Gets a New Liver* (Louisville, KY: Bridge Resources, 1997).

27. Arthur Caplan, "Sounding Board: Ethical and Policy Issues in the Procurement of Cadaver Organs for Transplantation," *New England Journal of Medicine* 311 (1984): 982–83.

28. For an argument that required request laws have not succeeded see M. K. Gaedeke Norris, "Required Request: Why It Has Not Significantly Improved the Donor Shortage," *Heart & Lung* 19 (1990): 685–86. For survey evidence that donor families find donation helpful in dealing with their loss, see Helen Levine Batten and Jeffrey Prottas, "Kind Strangers: The Families of Organ Donors," *Health Affairs* 6 (1987): 35–47. In addition to these changes, OPOs have become increasingly professionalized and have accumulated specialized knowledge about how to intervene. See Bonnie Harris Sammons, "Organ Recovery Coordinators Can Help Family Work through the Grieving Process," *AORN Journal* 48 (1988): 181–182; Julie Mull Strange and David Taylor, "Organ and Tissue donation," in *Transplantation Nursing: Acute and Long-Term Management,* ed. Marie T. Nolan and Sharon M. Augustine, 77–108 (Norwalk: Appleton & Lange, 1991); Barbara A. Helene Williams, Kathleen L. Grady, and Doris M. Sadiford-Guttenbeil, *Organ Transplantation: A Manual for Nurses* (New York: Springer, 1991); United Network for Organ Sharing, *UNOS Organ Procurement Coordinator's Handbook* (Richmond, VA: UNOS, 1995) and *Donation & Transplantation: Nursing Curriculum* (Richmond, VA: UNOS, n.d.).

29. To guard against this, there is a long-standing professional separation between the doctors who declare a patient dead and the transplant teams that harvest the organs. For a detailed discussion of the concept of brain death, see Richard M. Zaner, editor, *Death: Beyond Whole-Brain Criteria* (Boston: Kluwer Academic Publishers, 1988). The best recent discussion of the relationship between changing definitions of brain death and attitudes toward organ transplantation can be found in Lock, *Twice Dead.*

30. Abraham Twersky, Michael Gold, and Walter Jacob, "Jewish Perspectives," in *New Harvest: Transplanting the Body and Reaping the Benefits,* ed. C. Don Keyes and Walter E. Wiest (Clifton, NJ: Humana Press, 1991) p. 190. The halacha is the accumulated body of law and ethics in Orthodox Judaism. See also "Organ Transplant: Soon It May Be a Routine Part of the Jewish Death Ritual," *Jewish Voice,* December 1996.

31. Some churches oppose the harvesting of fetal tissue and organs for medical use, as the fetuses involved will normally have been aborted or grown in a test tube.

32. Raymond L. Horton and Patricia J. Horton, "Knowledge Regarding Organ Donation: Identifying and Overcoming Barriers to Organ Donation," *Social Science and Medicine* 31 (1990): 791–800.

33. United Network for Organ Sharing, *Organ and Tissue Donation: A Reference Guide for Clergy*, 3rd ed. (Richmond, VA: UNOS, 1998).

34. "Pope Warns of Danger in Organ Transplants and Genetic Testing," *New York Times,* October 27, 1980, A1.

35. The early ambivalence about organ transplants is reflected in the shifting emphasis of comments from the Vatican in the 1970s and early 1980s. John Paul II's worries were shared to some degree by his predecessor, but in his only statement on organ transplants John Paul I emphasized the benefits: "We are content today to express to you our congratulations and our trust, for the immense work that you put in the service of human life in order to prolong it in better conditions. The whole problem is to act with respect for the person and for one's neighbors, whether it is a question of donors of organs or beneficiaries, and never to transform man into an object of experiment." Frank Veith, "Organ Transplants and the Pope's Statement" (letter to the editor), *New York Times,* November 10, 1980, A22.

36. Batten and Prottas, "Kind Strangers," 35–47.

37. This idea can never be entirely symbolic, since the recipient does carry a physical piece of the donor alive inside them. There are also much stronger versions of it: In her memoir *A Change of Heart,* Claire Sylvia claims that after her heart-lung transplant she developed personality traits—including new tastes in food and clothes—that she later discovered were characteristic of the eighteen-year-old man her new organs came from. Claire Sylvia, *A Change of Heart: A Memoir* (New York: Little, Brown, 1997). Stories like this are a common part of popular culture about organ transplants.

38. Quotes are from notes on a talk given by Jack Locicero at Princeton University, April 20, 1999.

39. Pekkanen, *Donor,* 213.

40. Maria Banevicius, "An Investigation of Cadaver Organ Donor Families Three Years After Donation: A Pilot Study," master's thesis, Yale University School of Nursing, 1992, 35.

41. Banevicius, "Cadaver Organ Donor Families," 36.

42. Victoria Poole, *Thursday's Child* (New York: Little, Brown, 1980), 257.

43. Banevicius, "Cadaver Organ Donor Families," 38.

44. Kimbrell, *The Human Body Shop,* 30.

45. Arthur Caplan and Daniel Coelho, eds., *The Ethics of Organ Transplants* (Amherst: Prometheus Books, 1998), 11.

46. Espeland and Stevens, "Commensuration as a Social Process," pp. 313–43.

47. Zelizer, *Social Meaning of Money.*

48. Blair and Kaserman, "Economics and Ethics," 421. See also David Kaserman and A. H. Barnett, *The U.S. Organ Procurement System: A Prescription for Reform* (Washington, DC: American Enterprise Institute Press, 2002).

49. Hansmann, "Economics and Ethics," 57-85.

50. Lloyd Cohen, "Increasing the Supply of Transplant Organs: The Virtues of a Futures Market," *George Washington Law Review* 58 (1989): 1-51.

51. Sheryl Gay Stolberg, "Pennsylvania Set to Break Taboo On Reward for Organ Donations," *New York Times,* May 6, 1999, A1. See also Peter Ubel et al., "Pennsylvania's Voluntary Benefits Program: Evaluating an Innovative Proposal for Increasing Organ Donation," *Health Affairs* 19, no. 5 (2000): 206-11.

52. Christoper Snowbeck, "Organ Donor Funeral Aid Scrapped," *Pittsburgh Post Gazette,* February 1, 2002, B1.

53. Over the period of the sample, horror stories about organs-for-cash do persist, but become almost exclusively concerned with foreign reports of organ sales, particularly from India, South America and Southeast Asia. These stories are excluded from the data in Figure 2.3.

54. Charles Tilly, "Power—Top Down and Bottom Up," *Journal of Political Philosophy* 7 (1999): 341.

55. Radin, *Contested Commodities.*

56. The mistaken idea that market versus nonmarket exchange neatly lines up with renewable vs nonrenewable body parts probably persists because many people wrongly believe that there is for-profit blood collection in the United States. In fact, almost all of the whole blood collected is freely donated. There is a market for plasma, which complicates the issue. But this only reinforces the point: there is no convenient biological divide that maps onto the social organization of exchange.

57. See Radin, *Contested Commodities,* 79-101, for a discussion of the relationship between market rhetoric and commodification proper. As Peter Bearman notes, although the frontstage/backstage metaphor is a very useful way to analyze many social settings, there is no reason to believe a priori that the cynical rhetoric heard in backstage areas is any more "authentic, revelatory of personality, deep, honest or natural" than what happens in frontstage areas: it, too, is a performance. Peter Bearman, *Doormen* (Chicago: University of Chicago Press, 2005), 2.

58. "We have had some fabulous gifts. . . . We have had donors sent on cruises, we have had a year of tuition paid. The donor doesn't know what the gift is going to be. She just knows that there will be a gift, so that way she's still giving her eggs without undue compensation or any form of bribery." So says Teri Royal of the Options Egg Donor Agency, quoted in Rebecca Mead, "Eggs for Sale," *New Yorker,* August 9, 1999, 62.

59. David K. Cooper and Robert P. Lanza, *Xeno: The Promise of Transplanting Animal Organs into Humans* (New York: Oxford University Press, 2000).

60. In the last twenty-five years or so, bioethics has become the dominant arena in which to ask and answer questions about commodification. As a profession, it has expanded since the 1970s, staking its claim to authoritatively analyze these problems. This growth has not been uncontested. Rather, it seems to have been the outcome of a professional power struggle conducted

through the 1970s and '80s between scientists and theologians over who was the legitimate moral authority on these issues. See Evans, *Playing God?*; Charles L. Bosk, "Professional Ethicist Available: Logical, Secular, Friendly," *Dædalus* 128, no. 4 (1999): 47–68.

61. See, for instance, Zaner, *Death;* James F. Childress, "Ethical Criteria for Procuring and Distributing Organs for Transplantation," *Journal of Health Politics, Policy and Law* 14 (1989): 87–113; Larry R. Churchill and Rosa Lynn Pinkus, "The Use of Anencephalic Organs: Historical and Ethical Dimensions," *Milbank Quarterly* 68 (1990): 147–169; David Lamb, *Organ Transplants and Ethics* (New York: Routledge, 1990).

62. Arthur Caplan, *If I Were a Rich Man, Could I Buy a Pancreas?* (Indiana: Indiana University Press, 1994).

63. Anderson, *Value in Ethics and Economics;* Radin, *Contested Commodities;* Sunstein, *Free Markets and Social Justice.*

CHAPTER THREE

1. Liver, pancreas, and even lung transplants are now also possible using living donors. Lobes from the liver and lung can be removed from living patients and used for transplant, as can islet cells from pancreases. Transplants of this sort make up a small but increasing proportion of living-donor transplants.

2. Lock, "Deadly Disputes"; Hogle, *Recovering the Nation's Body.*

3. Gallup Organization, "The American Public's Attitudes toward Organ Donation and Transplantation: A Survey Conducted for the Partnership for Organ Donation" (Boston, February 1993). Support for organ donation also rises with education. The consensus among medical researchers (who do not always control for education when analyzing data on support for donation) is that the race gap in donation is large and persistent. See B. L. Kasiske et al., "The Effect of Race on Access and Outcome in Transplantation," *New England Journal of Medicine* 324 (1991): 320–27; M. Rozon-Solomon and L. Burrows, "'Tis Better to Receive Than to Give: The Relative Failure of the African American Community to Provide Organs for Transplantation," *Mount Sinai Journal of Medicine* 66, no. 4 (1999): 273–76; E. Guadagnoli et al., "The Influence of Race on Approaching Families for Organ Donation and Their Decision to Donate," *American Journal of Public Health* 89, no. 2 (1999): 244–47.

4. If we cross-classify the responses to these questions, we find that even the people who believed kidney sales should be allowed overwhelmingly chose first-come, first-served allocation of organs. In other words, a production market is partly endorsed, but not a consumer market.

5. Jeffrey Prottas, *The Most Useful Gift: Altruism and the Public Policy of Organ Transplants* (San Francisco: Jossey Bass, 1994).

6. OPOs may have quite different policies on this matter, however, as will be discussed below. See Dave Wendler and Neal Dickert, "The Consent Process for Cadaveric Organ Procurement: How Does It Work? How Can It Be

Improved?" *Journal of the American Medical Association* 285, no. 3 (2001): 329–33.

7. Peter Ubel and Arthur Caplan, "Geographic Favoritism in Liver Transplantation—Unfortunate or Unfair?" *New England Journal of Medicine* 339, no. 18 (1998): 1322–25.

8. Institute of Medicine, *Organ Procurement and Transplantation* (Washington, DC: National Academy Press, 1999).

9. For further discussion of the question of organ allocation, see Michael J. Dennis, "Scarce Medical Resources: Hemodialysis and Kidney Transplantation," in *Local Justice in America,* ed. Jon Elster, 81–152 (New York: Russell Sage Foundation, 1995).

10. General Accounting Office, *Organ Procurement Organizations: Alternatives Being Developed to More Accurately Assess Performance* (Washington, DC: General Accounting Office, 1997), GAO/HEHS-98-26.

11. Cancer, AIDS, and heart disease are causes of death that may rule out procurement of some or all organs. A body's not being found for a month after death would have the same effect.

12. GAO, *Organ Procurement Organizations,* 22.

13. Imagine x, y, and z are three proposed measures of a single underlying variable. A priori, we have reason to believe that x is a less accurate measure than y and y is a less accurate measure than z. It will be easier for an OPO to score a "passing grade" on x than on y and on y than on z. We then check to see how many OPOs get a passing grade on each measure. To be confident that the three measures were tapping one underlying variable with differing accuracy, rather than three different underlying variables, we would want to observe that (1) every OPO that failed x failed y, and every one that failed y failed z; (2) every OPO that passed z passed y, and every one that passed y passed x. This is the pattern that the GAO found for the three measures discussed in the text.

14. Roberta G. Simmons, "Altruism and Sociology," *Sociological Quarterly* 32 (1991): 3.

15. Elliot Sober and David Sloan Wilson, *Unto Others: The Evolution and Psychology of Unselfish Behavior* (Cambridge, MA: Harvard University Press, 1998), 228.

16. Alan Wolfe, "What Is Altruism?," in *Private Action and the Public Good,* ed. Walter W. Powell and Elisabeth S. Clemens, 36–46 (New Haven: Yale University Press, 1998).

17. Sober and Wilson, *Unto Others,* 17.

18. David Schmidtz, "Reasons for Altruism," *Social Philosophy and Policy* 10, no. 1 (1993): 65.

19. The classic results are in W. D. Hamilton, "The Genetical Evolution of Social Behavior," pts. 1 and 2, *Journal of Theoretical Biology* 7 (1964): 1–16, 17–52, and J. Maynard Smith, "Group Selection and Kin Selection," *Nature* 201 (1964): 1145–46. More ambitiously, Sober and Wilson's *Unto Others* argues that multilevel or group-selection mechanisms may favor the evolution of altruism in

populations to a greater degree than has generally been accepted by biologists. R. L. Trivers, "The Evolution of Reciprocal Altruism," *Quarterly Review of Biology* 46 (1971): 35–57, defines the concept of reciprocal altruism, later developed in Robert Axelrod and W. D. Hamilton, "The Evolution of Cooperation," *Science* 211 (1981): 1390–96; John Maynard Smith, *Evolution and the Theory of Games* (New York: Cambridge University Press, 1982); and Robert Axelrod, *The Evolution of Cooperation* (New York: Basic Books, 1984). The "tit-for-tat" strategy (invented by Anatol Rapoport and described in Axelrod's *The Evolution of Cooperation)* is often said not to be altruistic, because the cooperator benefits in the long run. There is some disagreement about this: Sober and Wilson (*Unto Others,* 84) argue that the distinction is not built into a formal model of these processes but lies instead in their interpretation. Other studies show how altruistic and cooperative behavior can be transmitted by cultural means, sometimes using cultural analogs of the kin- or group-selection mechanisms. These include Paul Allison, "The Cultural Evolution of Beneficial Norms," *Social Forces* 71 (1992), 279–301; Robert Boyd and Peter J. Richerson, *Culture and the Evolutionary Process* (Chicago: University of Chicago Press, 1985); Michael Macy and John Skvoretz, "The Evolution of Trust and Cooperation between Strangers: A Computational Model," *American Sociological Review* 63 (1998): 638–60; and Noah Mark, "The Cultural Evolution of Cooperation," *American Sociological Review* 67, no. 3 (2002): 323–44.

20. Jane Allyn Piliavin and Hong-Wen Charng, "Altruism: A Review of Recent Theory and Research," *Annual Review of Sociology* 16 (1990): 29.

21. M. L. Hoffman, "Is Altruism Part of Human Nature?" *Journal of Personality and Social Psychology* 40 (1981): 121–37; C. D. Batson, "Prosocial Motivation: Is It Ever Truly Altruistic?" in *Advances in Experimental Social Psychology,* vol. 20, ed. L. Berkowitz, 65–122 (New York: Academic Press, 1987); Piliavin and Callero, *Giving Blood.*

22. Gallup, "American Public's Attitudes"; Prottas, *Most Useful Gift.*

23. J. Shanteau and R. Harris, eds., *Organ Donation and Transplantation: Psychological and Behavioral Factors* (Washington, DC: APA Press, 1990).

24. B. Latané and J. M. Darley, "Social Determinants of Bystander Intervention in Emergencies," in *Altruism and Helping Behavior: Social Psychological Studies of Some Antecedents and Consequences,* ed. J. Macaulay and L. Berkowitz, 13–27 (New York: Academic Press, 1970); W. Austin, "Sex Differences in Bystander Intervention in a Theft," *Journal of Personality and Social Psychology* 37 (1979): 2110–20; D. K. Krebs and D. T. Miller, "Altruism and Aggression," in *Handbook of Social Psychology,* 3rd ed., ed. G. Lindzey and E. Aronson, 2:1–71 (New York: Random House, 1985).

25. Simmons, "Altruism and Sociology," 5.

26. Piliavin and Charng, "Altruism," 58.

27. Paul G. Schervish and John J. Havens, "Social Participation and Charitable Giving: A Multivariate Analysis," *Voluntas* 8 (1997): 235–60.

28. Peter Frumkin, *On Being Nonprofit: A Conceptual and Policy Primer* (Cambridge, MA: Harvard University Press, 2002), 102.

29. Lee Clarke and Carroll Estes, "Sociological and Economic Theories of Markets and Nonprofits: Evidence from Home Health Organizations," *American Journal of Sociology* 97 (1992): 945–69; Victoria Alexander, "Environmental Constraints and Organizational Strategies," in *Private Action and the Public Good,* ed. Walter W. Powell and Elisabeth S. Clemens, 272–90 (New Haven: Yale University Press, 1998); Kirsten Grønbjerg, *Understanding Nonprofit Funding: Managing Revenues in Social Service and Community Development Organizations* (San Francisco: Jossey-Bass, 1993); Christine Oliver, "Strategic Responses to Institutional Processes," *Academy of Management Review* 16 (1991): 145–79; Emily Barman, "Asserting Difference: The Strategic Response of Nonprofit Organizations to Competition," *Social Forces* 80 (2002): 1191–1222.

30. Simmons, Marine, and Simmons, *Gift of Life.*

31. D. Zimmerman et al., "Gender Disparity in Living Renal Transplant Donation," *American Journal of Kidney Diseases* 36, no. 3 (2000): 534–40.

32. Margaret Verble and Judy Worth, "Overcoming Families' Fears and Concerns in the Donation Discussion," *Progress in Transplantation* 10, no. 3 (2000): 155–60; R. N. Ehrle, T. J. Shafer, and K. R. Nelson, "Referral, Request and Consent for Organ Donation: Best Practice—A Blueprint for Success," *Critical Care Nurse* 19 (1999): 21–33; Gortmaker, "Improving the Request Process," 210–17.

33. There have not been many studies of the procurement rate, as distinct from studies of dispositions to donate. Prottas suggests five measures of OPO effectiveness: referrals of potential donors per capita, consent rate of donor families, kidney and nonrenal organs donated per capita, and the rate of kidneys discarded. Jeffrey Prottas, "The Organization of Organ Procurement," *Journal of Health Politics, Policy and Law* 14, no. 1 (1989): 41–55. The measure used here is more accurate than a per capita measure for reasons discussed in the text. National data on consent rates are not available. The kidney discard rate is a useful measure: it tells us the percentage of kidneys procured by an OPO that end up being unsuitable for use. In 1997, this number averaged about 11 percent, with a high of more than 38 percent. The discard rate was not correlated with the procurement rate ($r = -0.007$). Using a per million population measure, Evans, Orians, and Ascher argued that OPOs were not turning potential donors into actual donors. Their analysis suggested that the number of donors in the United States could be increased by 80 percent. R. Evans, C. Orians, and N. Ascher, "The Potential Supply of Organ Donors," *Journal of the American Medical Association* 267, no. 2 (1992): 239–46. Similarly, Christiansen et al. estimated that actual donations were between 28 and 44 percent of the potential total in the regions they studied. C. L. Christiansen et al., "A Method for Estimating Solid Organ Donor Potential by Organ Procurement Region," *American Journal of Public Health* 88, no. 11 (1998): 1645–50. However, Siminoff and Nelson, when they carried out a microlevel review

of hospital chart data in one OPO region, found that it is easy to overestimate the number of potential donors based on standard reporting procedures. Laura Siminoff and Kristine Nelson, "The Accuracy of Hospital Reports of Organ Donation Eligibility, Requests and Consent: A Cross-Validation Study," *Joint Commission Journal on Quality Improvement* 25, no. 3 (1999): 129–36. In 1992, the General Accounting Office surveyed all OPOs in an effort to determine whether some OPOs' performance was subpar; it collected data on procurement rates but did not examine the question of what predicted procurement. General Accounting Office, *Organ Transplants: Increased Effort Needed to Boost Supply and Ensure Equitable Distribution of Organs,* 1993, GAO/HRD-93-56. Finally, a mail survey of OPOs was carried out in 1995 with the intent of finding which were efficient and which were inefficient. Although it measured a number of organizational characteristics, this study did not control for variability in the characteristics of OPO service areas. Y. A. Ozcan, J. W. Begun, and M. M. McKinney, "Benchmarking Organ Procurement Organizations: A National Study," *Health Services Research* 34, no. 4 (1999): 855–74.

34. Ehrle, Shafer, and Nelson, "Referral, Request and Consent," 21–33; J. E. Kopfman et al., "Influence of Race on Cognitive and Affective Reactions to Organ Donation Messages," *Transplantation Proceedings* 34 (2002): 3035–41; Gallup, "American Public's Attitudes."

35. Margaret Verble et al., "A Multiethnic Study of the Relationship between Fears and Concerns and Refusal Rates," *Progress in Transplantation* 12, no. 3 (2002): 185–90; Verble and Worth, "Overcoming Families' Fears."

36. Kasiske et al., "Effect of Race"; V. R. Randall, "Slavery, Segregation and Racism: Trusting the Medical System Ain't Always Easy! An African-American Perspective on Bioethics," *St. Louis University Public Law Review* 15 (1996): 181–235; S. L. Gortmaker, "Organ Donor Potential and Performance: Size and Nature of the Organ Donor Shortfall," *Critical Care Medicine* 24 (1996): 432–39.

37. Rozon-Solomon and Burrows, "'Tis Better to Receive."

38. J. Z. Ayanian et al., "The Effect of Patients' Preferences on Racial Differences in Access to Renal Transplantation," *New England Journal of Medicine* 341, no. 22 (1999): 1661–69; Kasiske et al., "Effect of Race." This is also true of women and the poor. See G. C. Alexander and A. R. Seghal, "Barriers to Cadaveric Renal Transplantation among Blacks, Women, and the Poor," *Journal of the American Medical Association* 280, no. 13 (1998): 1148–52.

39. Gallup, "American Public's Attitudes"; Southeastern Institute of Research, "General Consumers: American Attitudes toward the Allocation of Organ Transplantation" (Richmond, VA: United Network for Organ Sharing, 1994).

40. M. D. Jendrisak et al., "Cadaveric-Donor Organ Recovery at a Hospital-Independent Facility," *Transplantation* 74, no. 7 (2002): 931–32.

41. A. C. Klassen et al., "Organizational Characteristics of Solid-Organ Donor Hospitals and Nondonor Hospitals," *Journal of Transplant Coordination* 9 (1999): 87–94.

42. Ann C. Klassen and David K. Klassen, "Who Are the Donors in Organ Donation? The Family's Perspective in Mandated Choice," *Annals of Internal Medicine* 125 (1996): 70–73.

43. Laura Siminoff et al., "Factors Influencing Families' Consent for Donation of
Solid Organs for Transplantation," *Journal of the American Medical Association*
286, no. 1 (July 4, 2001): 71–77; Verble et al., "Multiethnic Study."

44. Wolfe, "What Is Altruism?"; Mark Schlesinger, "Mismeasuring the Consequences of Ownership: External Influences and the Comparative Performance of Public, For-Profit, and Private Nonprofit Organizations," in *Private
Action and the Public Good,* ed. Walter W. Powell and Elisabeth S. Clemens, 85–
113 (New Haven: Yale University Press, 1998); V. Hodgkinson and M. Weitzman, *Giving and Volunteering in the United States: Findings from a National
Survey* (Washington, DC: Independent Sector, 1992); Piliavin and Charng,
"Altruism."

45. David J. Powner and Joseph M. Darby, "Current Considerations in the Issue of
Brain Death," *Neurosurgery* 45 (1999) : 1225.

46. Wendler and Dickert, "Consent Process for Cadaveric Organ Procurement."

47. Wendler and Dickert asked representatives of OPOs how likely their organizations would be (in the abstract) to procure organs in circumstances where
either (1) the potential donor left a record of her wish to donate but the next
of kin opposed donation or (2) the next of kin favored donation but the
potential donor had left a record of his wish not to donate. The survey also
varied the strength of the potential donor's support for or objection to donation: from repeated verbal statements before death, through a signed or
unsigned donor card, to designated durable power of attorney. OPO
responses varied considerably. We can use this data to measure how willing
an OPO may be to procure organs even under difficult circumstances.
This is not an ideal measure of actual practice, for which no data are available. Nevertheless, respondents were very knowledgeable about the procurement process: "A total of 26 (43 percent) respondents were the OPOs'
executive directors, 19 (31 percent) were procurement or organ recovery
coordinators, 11 (18 percent) were directors of procurement, and 5 (8 percent) were chief executive officers. A total of 51 (84 percent) had been
employed by their current OPO for 3 or more years, and 41 (67 percent) had
been employed by their current OPO for more than 6 years" (Wendler and
Dickert, "Consent Process for Cadaveric Organ Procurement," 331).

48. In an otherwise identical model with donors per million population as the
dependent variable, the education effect is stronger and more significantly
negative than reported in table A.1. In such a model, we can interpret the
coefficient as measuring the contribution of education to circumstance of
death.

49. The details in this paragraph are drawn from Robert M. Sade et al., "Increasing Organ Donation: A Successful New Concept," *Transplantation* 72 (2002):
1142–46.

50. Sade et al., "Increasing Organ Donation," 1144.

51. Evan Schofer and Marion Fourcade-Gourinchas, "The Structural Contexts of Civic Engagement: Voluntary Association Membership in Comparative Perspective," *American Sociological Review* 66 (2001): 806–28, 807. See also Theda Skocpol, Marshal Ganz, and Ziah Munson, "A Nation of Organizers: The Institutional Origins of Civic Voluntarism in the United States," *American Political Science Review* 94 (2000): 527–46, and Lester M. Salamon and Helmut K. Anheier, *The Nonprofit Sector in Comparative Perspective: An Overview* (Baltimore: Johns Hopkins University Press, 1994).

CHAPTER FOUR

1. Elster, "Selfishness and Altruism," 40.

2. See, for example, Radin, *Contested Commodities,* 96; Amitai Etzioni, *The Moral Dimension: Toward a New Economics* (New York: Free Press, 1988), 75; Walzer, *Spheres of Justice,* 91.

3. J. A. Piliavin, "Why Do They Give the Gift of Life? A Review of Research on Blood Donors since 1977," *Transfusion* 30 (1990): 444–59.

4. R. M. Oswalt, "A Review of Blood Donor Motivation and Recruitment," *Transfusion* 17 (1977): 123–35; Piliavin, "Why Do They Give?"

5. R. D. Roberts and M. D. Wolkoff, "Improving the Quality of Whole-Blood Supply: Limits to Voluntary Arrangements," *Journal of Health Policy, Politics and Law* 13 (1988): 167–78.

6. Piliavin and Callero, *Giving Blood.*

7. Piliavin, "Why Do They Give?"; Oswalt, "Review of Blood Donor Motivation"; R. M. Oswalt and T. E. Hoff, "The Motivations of Blood Donors and Non-Donors: A Community Survey," *Transfusion* 15 (1975): 68–72; P. London and B. M. Hemphill, "The Motivations of Blood Donors," *Transfusion* 14 (1965): 559–68.

8. A. W. Drake, S. N. Finkelstein, and H. M. Sapolsky, *The American Blood Supply* (Cambridge, MA: MIT Press, 1982), 81–83.

9. Titmuss, *Gift Relationship.*

10. Karlheinz Reif and Eric Marlier, *Eurobarometer 41.0* (Ann Arbor: Inter-University Consortium for Political Research, 1995).

11. Piet Hagen, *Blood Transfusion in Europe: A White Paper* (Strasbourg: Council of Europe, 1993); W. G. van Aken, *The Collection and Use of Human Blood and Plasma in Europe* (Strasbourg: Council of Europe, 1993); Bernard Genetet, *Blood Transfusion: Half a Century of Contribution by the Council of Europe* (Strasbourg: Council of Europe, 1998).

12. Hagen, *Blood Transfusion in Europe,* 34ff. Unless otherwise cited, information in the following paragraphs comes from this source.

13. Germany is the only such "mixed" system where the Red Cross holds a majority. It is an unusual case in other respects also. First, as of 1989 it was the only European Union country that obtained some of its blood from paid suppliers.

Second, there is a mixed system of paid and unpaid donation within the non-profit sector. Most hospital and community blood banks pay between 30 and 50 DM (about $18 to $30) per donation. (Government policy stipulates a 50 DM maximum.) In some areas Red Cross collection centers also compensate their donors. Third, regional governments (the various *Länder*) have different collection policies. There are also significant differences between eastern and western *Länder*.

14. Hagen, *Blood Transfusion in Europe,* 58.
15. Interesting given this apparently strong volunteer activity is the charge that Italy does not have a large voluntary sector. See, for example, Ted Perlmutter, "Italy: Why No Voluntary Sector?" in *Between States and Markets: The Voluntary Sector in Comparative Perspective,* ed. Robert Wuthnow, 157–88 (Princeton: Princeton University Press, 1991).
16. There is only a weak positive correlation between giving blood and giving money or time. See Lee, Piliavin, and Call, "Giving Time, Money and Blood."
17. Andrew Greeley, "The Other Civic America: Religion and Social Capital," *American Prospect* 32 (1997): 68–73.
18. Greeley, "Other Civic America," 71.
19. Wuthnow, *Acts of Compassion;* Mark Chaves, "The Religious Ethic and the Spirit of Nonprofit Entrepreneurship," in *Private Action and the Public Good,* ed. Walter W. Powell and Elisabeth S. Clemens, 47–68 (New Haven: Yale University Press, 1998).
20. C. Clotfelter, "On Trends in Private Sources of Support for the US Non-profit Sector," *Voluntas* 4, no. 2 (1993): 190–95; Hodgkinson and Weitzman, *Giving and Volunteering;* Christopher Jencks, "Who Gives to What?" in *The Nonprofit Sector: A Research Handbook,* ed. Walter W. Powell, 331–39 (New Haven: Yale University Press, 1992).
21. Hodgkinson and Weitzman, *Giving and Volunteering;* Piliavin and Charng, "Altruism."
22. Drake, Finkelstein, and Sapolsky, *American Blood Supply,* 76–113.
23. Table A.3 shows the results from a series of logistic regressions in which seven individual-level variables were regressed on the donor variable (had the respondent ever given blood) for each country in the sample. The model tests predictions about individual donors and also gives a sense of the range of cross-national variation in the donor profile.
24. A significant gap persists in Ireland, Germany, Italy, Portugal, and Luxembourg.
25. I recalculated the rates reported in Greeley, "Other Civic America," using an EVS survey question that asked the respondent if they did unpaid work for one of sixteen kinds of voluntary organization, ranging from church organizations and trade unions to sports, animal rights, community action, and other groups. The volunteering rate is the proportion of the population that did unpaid work for at least one of these activities. It ranges from a low of 7.6 per cent in Spain to a high of 35.6 per cent in Norway. The comparable statistic for the United States (from the same survey wave) is 47 per cent.

26. The correlation coefficient is –0.004.
27. The correlation coefficient is 0.81. The corresponding correlations for the other regimes are $r = 0.28$ (for state systems) and $r = -0.13$ (for blood banks).
28. The model specification is discussed in more detail in the appendix. The results of the analysis are reported there in table A.4, and figure 4.3 below is derived from those estimates.
29. See Rene Bekkers, *Giving and Volunteering in the Netherlands: Sociological and Psychological Perspectives* (Amsterdam: Thesis Publishers (Utrecht University), 2004) for a study of the Netherlands, for example.

CHAPTER FIVE

1. Carol Heimer, "Allocating Information Costs in a Negotiated Information Order: Interorganizational Constraints on Decision Making in Norwegian Oil Insurance," *Administrative Science Quarterly* 30 (1985): 395–417.
2. Titmuss, *Gift Relationship.*
3. H. M. Sapolsky and S. N. Finkelstein, "Blood Policy Revisited—A New Look at the Gift Relationship," *Public Interest* 46 (1977): 15–27.
4. Institute of Medicine, *HIV and the Blood Supply: An Analysis of Crisis Decision-making* (Washington, DC: National Academy Press, 1995), 41.
5. Viviana Zelizer, "Beyond the Polemics of the Market: Establishing a Theoretical and Empirical Agenda," *Sociological Forum* 3 (1988): 622.
6. For early criticism of Titmuss on this point, see Sapolsky and Finkelstein, "Blood Policy Revisited," 15–27; A. J. Culyer, "Blood and Altruism: An Economic Review," in *Blood Policy: Issues and Alternatives,* ed. David B. Johnson, 29–58 (Washington, DC: American Enterprise Institute for Public Policy Research, 1976); and Reuben Kessel, "Transfused Blood, Serum Hepatitis and the Coase Theorem," also in Johnson, *Blood Policy,* 183–207.
7. The hepatitis family has grown steadily since the 1960s. Hepatitis A, the mildest form, is spread orally. Although blood-borne transmission is possible, it is very rare. What Titmuss called serum hepatitis is caused by the hepatitis B virus, which is spread through the blood supply and is very infectious. It was discovered in 1965, and by 1968 a direct test (the hepatitis B surface antigen test) was available. A vaccine for HBV did not become available until 1982. In 1977, the hepatitis Delta virus was discovered. This is an incomplete RNA virus that can be transmitted only in the company of HBV. By the late 1970s, it became clear that there was still another form of hepatitis being transmitted through the blood supply. The virus causing this form was identified in 1989 and named hepatitis C.
8. Kessel, "Transfused Blood," 190.
9. Piliavin and Callero, *Giving Blood;* Hagen, *Blood Transfusion in Europe.*
10. Properly speaking, there are three kinds of organization and two representative bodies in this voluntary sector. The American Red Cross is the largest. Community blood banks operate on a smaller, local scale. Hospital blood banks collect blood for use only by their controlling hospital. The American

Association of Blood Banks and the Council of Community Blood Centers are the two representative groups. In the past, the Red Cross and the blood banks have had differing views about how blood should be collected. The Red Cross has always promoted a voluntary, community-based approach. The blood banks used to advocate a (sometimes for-profit) philosophy of individual responsibility but now hold a position much more like that of the Red Cross. In this chapter, references to blood banks refer also to the Red Cross.

11. IOM, *HIV and the Blood Supply,* 29.

12. IOM, *HIV and the Blood Supply,* 31.

13. Pamela Westfall, "Hepatitis, AIDS and the Blood Products Exemption from Strict Products Liability in California: A Reassessment," *Hastings Law Journal* 37 (1986): 1101–32. Note that if liability were to fall anywhere, it would be on the blood banks and plasma companies. This is true even though blood banks sell blood to and patients receive blood from hospitals. Hospitals may be liable for a whole variety of other risky interactions with patients, but the implicit contract for blood transfusions remains between the patient and the blood bank. This chapter does not discuss the relationship between hospitals and the blood banks, chiefly for want of information. I expect that, given that they are a captive market, hospitals do not play a very important a role in blood banks' calculations.

14. Jens Beckert, "What Is Sociological about Economic Sociology? Uncertainty and the Embeddedness of Economic Action," *Theory and Society* 25 (1996): 803–40.

15. For something of the former difficulty, see Charles Perrow and Mauro F. Guillen, *The AIDS Disaster* (New Haven: Yale University Press, 1990), and Sandra Panem, *The AIDS Bureaucracy* (Cambridge, MA: Harvard University Press, 1998). For the latter, see Randy Shilts, *And the Band Played On: Politics, People and the AIDS Epidemic* (New York: St Martin's Press, 1988), especially 115–16, 160–63, 168–71, and 220–26. Perrow and Guillen's valuable work is the only study of the blood supply from the perspective of the sociology of organizations. Shilts's book is the standard history of the period, but his focus is not on the blood suppliers as such. H. M. Sapolsky and S. L. Boswell, "The History of Transfusion AIDS: Practice and Policy Alternatives," in *AIDS: The Making of a Chronic Disease,* ed. Elizabeth Fee and Daniel M. Fox, 170–93 (Berkeley: University of California Press, 1992), characterize the structural differences between the blood banks and the plasma companies in an effort to explain their different reactions. They argue that the plasma companies reacted better because they were market-driven organizations with a competitive interest in selling a demonstrably safer product, whereas the blood banks wished merely to protect their quiet monopolies. This goes some of the way toward a satisfactory explanation. But Sapolsky and Boswell tend to argue for the general superiority of markets, much as Titmuss supported the opposite view.

16. For reviews see Carol Heimer, "Social Structure, Psychology and the Estimation of Risk," *Annual Review of Sociology* 14 (1988): 491–519, and Lee Clarke

and James F. Short, "Social Organization and Risk: Some Current Controversies," *Annual Review of Sociology* 19 (1993): 375–99.

17. Heimer, "Allocating Information Costs."

18. Heimer, "Allocating Information Costs," 398.

19. Heimer, "Allocating Information Costs," 397. See also Martha S. Feldman and James G. March, "Information in Organizations as Signal and Symbol," *Administrative Science Quarterly* 26 (1981): 171–86.

20. National Research Council archive of background material provided to the Institute of Medicine's Committee to Study HIV Transmission through Blood and Blood Products, Bruce Evatt interview notes, 1983 (box 2, folder 25), and transcript of Blood Products Advisory Council meeting, February 7–8, 1983 (box 3, tab 86).

21. Jeffrey Pfeffer and Gerald Salancik, *The External Dependence of Organizations: A Resource Dependence Perspective* (New York: Harper and Row, 1978).

22. Mark Granovetter, "Economic Action and Social Structure: The Problem of Embeddedness," *American Journal of Sociology* 91 (1985): 481–510.

23. If a voluntary organization can rely on a steady supply of contributions from the public, it will be structurally dependent on the recipients of its charity. The organization owes its existence to them. If the recipients no longer need help, then the charity is threatened with death regardless of the number of people willing to donate money to it. More often than not in such a situation, the organization finds a new group to assist. This is the well-known phenomenon of goal succession.

24. Information on the internal workings of these organizations comes largely from an archive held by the National Research Council. See the appendix for more on the data sources used for this chapter.

25. Piliavin and Callero, *Giving Blood,* 1.

26. IOM, *HIV and the Blood Supply,* 101–2, 104.

27. Shilts, *And the Band Played On,* 105.

28. At this time, HIV had yet to be discovered. The only way to test blood for the virus (assuming there was one) was to test it for surrogate markers, i.e., known items reliably found in the blood of AIDS patients. A hepatitis B core antigen test was the earliest such test. In early 1983, the CDC believed that implementing this test would detect 90 per cent of donors with AIDS. See IOM, *HIV and the Blood Supply,* 106.

29. NRC archive, Evatt interview notes."

30. IOM, *HIV and the Blood Supply,* 221.

31. IOM, *HIV and the Blood Supply,* 221.

32. NRC archive, June Osborn interview notes, 1994 (box 2, folder 25).

33. Mary Douglas, *Risk and Blame* (New York: Routledge, 1982), 22–37.

34. IOM, *HIV and the Blood Supply,* 106.

35. In autologous donation, a patient builds up a store of his or her own blood prior to surgery. Though categorized as a kind of donation, it obviously has no altruistic component. Autologous donations account for about 2 percent of the blood supply.

36. IOM, *HIV and the Blood Supply,* 277.

37. IOM, *HIV and the Blood Supply,* 285–89.

38. IOM, *HIV and the Blood Supply,* 285.

39. IOM, *HIV and the Blood Supply,* 111.

40. IOM, *HIV and the Blood Supply,* 287; emphasis in original.

41. NRC archive, transcript of BPAC meeting, February 7–8, 1983, 46.

42. NRC archive, transcript of BPAC meeting, February 7–8, 1983.

43. NRC archive, Joseph Bove interview notes, 1994 (box 2, folder 25).

44. IOM, *HIV and the Blood Supply,* 270.

45. IOM, *HIV and the Blood Supply* p. 93.

46. NRC archive, transcript of Blood Products Advisory Council meeting, December 4, 1982, 104.

47. IOM, *HIV and the Blood Supply,* 169–207.

48. IOM, *HIV and the Blood Supply,* 195–96.

49. IOM, *HIV and the Blood Supply,* 172.

50. IOM, *HIV and the Blood Supply,* 212.

51. IOM, *HIV and the Blood Supply,* 265; emphasis in original.

52. NRC archive, minutes of National Hemophilia Foundation meeting, October 22, 1983 (box 3).

53. For a full account of the swine flu case see Diana Dutton, *Worse Than the Disease* (New York: Cambridge University Press, 1988).

54. See the essays in Eric A. Feldman and Ronald Bayer, eds., *Blood Feuds: AIDS, Blood, and the Politics of Medical Disaster* (New York: Oxford University Press, 1999).

55. Paul Rabinow, *French DNA: Trouble in Purgatory* (Chicago: University of Chicago Press, 1999).

56. Starr, *Blood* p. 285–292.

57. Catherine Waldby et al., "Blood and Bioidentity: Ideas about Self, Boundaries and Risk among Blood Donors and People Living with Hepatitis C," *Social Science and Medicine* 59 (2004): 1461–71; M. Finucane, P. Slovic, and C. Mertz, "Public Perception of the Risk of Blood Transfusion," *Transfusion* 40 (2000): 1017–22.

58. J. P. O'Carroll, "Blood," in *Encounters with Modern Ireland,* ed. M. Peillon and E. Slater, 107–14 (Dublin: Institute of Public Administration, 1999); Ulrich Beck, *Risk Society* (London: Sage, 1992).

CHAPTER SIX

1. Michael Redfern, *The Royal Liverpool Children's Inquiry* (Liverpool: United Kingdom Department of Health, 2001).

2. United Kingdom Department of Health, *Report of a Census of Organs and Tissues Retained by Pathology Services in England* (London, 2000).

3. "The Return of the Bodysnatchers," *Economist,* February 3, 2001, 59–60. Organ procurement rates in the UK do appear to have fallen in recent years, though the decline began around 1995, prior to the Alder Hey scandal.

4. Glenys Spray, *Blood, Sweat and Tears: The Hepatitis C Scandal* (Dublin: Wolf-hound Press, 1998); T. Finlay, *Report of the Tribunal of Inquiry into the Blood Transfusion Service Board* (Dublin: Stationery Office, 1997).

5. Nick Madigan, "Inquiry Widens After 2 Arrests in Cadaver Case at UCLA," *New York Times,* March 9, 2004, A21.

6. Kimberly Edds, "UCLA Denies Role in Cadaver Case," *Washington Post,* March 9, 2004, A03.

7. See, for example, Stephen J. Hedges and William Gaines, "Donor Bodies Milled into Growing Profits," *Chicago Tribune,* May 21, 2000, A1, A16–17; William Heisel and Mark Katches, "Organ Agencies Aid For-Profit Suppliers," *Orange County Register,* June 25, 2000; Mark Katches and William Heisel, "Preliminary Tissue-Trade Report Issued," *Orange County Register,* August 9, 2000.

8. Hedges and Gaines, "Donor Bodies Milled into Growing Profits."

9. Office of Evaluation and Inspections, *Oversight of Tissue Banking* (Washington, DC: Department of Health and Human Services, 2001), OEI 01-00-00441.

10. O'Carroll, "Blood."

11. Scheper-Hughes, "Global Traffic in Human Organs"; Cohen, "Where It Hurts." Lock, *Twice Dead,* and Hogle, *Recovering the Nation's Body,* are important contributions to the cultural anthropology of donation in Western societies.

12. Evans, *Playing God?*

13. Pierre Bourdieu, *Practical Reason* (Stanford: Stanford University Press, 1998), 95; parentheses omitted, emphasis in the original.

14. Bourdieu, *Practical Reason,* 95.

15. The *habitus* is the set of dispositions and tendencies to behave in particular ways that people rely on to act in everyday life. For Bourdieu, it is a system of bodily habits of a semiautomatic character that provides people with templates for actions in both familiar and new social situations. Because our habitus emerges from the previous interactions we have had—encounters that themselves took place in particular class and cultural contexts shaped by the habits and dispositions of others—it has a durable and systematic quality that reflects the wider social structure and enables that structure to be continually and actively reproduced in everyday life.

16. Bourdieu, *Practical Reason,* 97.

17. See Elster, *Sour Grapes;* Jon Elster, *Ulysses and the Sirens* (New York: Cambridge University Press, 1984).

18. Bourdieu, *Practical Reason,* 98. A third possibility is to argue that, by following some simple local rules, the members of a society are reproducing a social structure that they are aware of in practice but whose general structure they cannot articulate. Peter Bearman gives a convincing illustration of this approach in his analysis of the marriage practices of a small group of Australian aboriginals, who were originally studied in the 1940s. He is able to identify a stable pattern of marriage exchanges between eleven blocks of the social structure, blocks that do not map onto any of the cultural categories of

the social group (such as tribal or totemic identities). Members of the society could identify marriages that violated the underlying exchange pattern, even though they could not really say how they knew this, and neither could they articulate the general rules governing the exchange structure. This kind of practical knowledge is a plausible solution to the problem of how some kinds of social patterns get reproduced in an apparently self-sustaining way. It would apply more directly to our case if it were not already clear that the nature of gifts is the subject of considerable discursive elaboration in both tribal and modern socieites. See Peter Bearman, "Generalized Exchange," *American Journal of Sociology* 102 (1997): 1383–1415.

19. Bourdieu, *Practical Reason,* 98.
20. Titmuss, *Gift Relationship,* 306.
21. Banevicius, "Cadaver Organ Donor Families."
22. Courtney Bender, *Heaven's Kitchen: Living Religion at God's Love We Deliver* (Chicago: University of Chicago Press, 2003).
23. Studying a small town in the late 1970s, Theodore Caplow found that everyone participated in Christmas gift giving, but exchanges were almost exclusively confined to kin rather than friendship networks. It would be interesting to know whether this remains true. See Theodore Caplow, "Christmas Gifts and Kin Networks," *American Sociological Review* 47 (1982) pp. 383–392.
24. Hochschild, *Managed Heart.*
25. Roger Friedland and Robert R. Alford, "Bringing Society Back In: Symbols, Practices and Institutional Contradictions," in *The New Institutionalism and Organizational Analysis,* ed. Walter Powell and Paul DiMaggio, 232–66 (Chicago: University of Chicago Press, 1991).
26. Sade et al., "Increasing Organ Donation."
27. Erving Goffman, "On Cooling the Mark Out: Some Aspects of Adaptation to Failure," *Psychiatry* 15 (1952): 451–63.
28. O'Neill, *Autonomy and Trust,* 156.
29. Albert Hirschman, *The Passions and the Interests* (Princeton: Princeton University Press, 1978).
30. Allan Silver, "Friendship in Commercial Society: Eighteenth-Century Social Theory and Modern Sociology," *American Journal of Sociology* 95, no. 6 (1990): 1474–1504.
31. For a review see Matthew Rabin, "Psychology and Economics," *Journal of Economic Literature* 36 (1998): 11–46.
32. Joseph Henrich et al., "In Search of Homo Economicus: Behavioral Experiments in 15 Small-Scale Societies," *American Economic Review* 91 (2001): 76–77.
33. Jonathan Parry, "The Gift, the Indian Gift and the 'Indian Gift'," *Man* 21 (1986) p. 466. This conception of the gift is better thought of as a present, rather than a gift in the Maussian sense.
34. Carrier, "Gifts, Commodities and Social Relations," 125–26.

35. Espeland and Stevens, "Commensuration as a Social Process"; Carruthers and Stinchcombe, "Social Structure of Liquidity."

36. A very useful analysis of this issue, which I follow here, is given by Allen W. Wood, "Exploitation," *Social Philosophy and Policy* 12, no. 2 (1995): 136–58.

37. Wood, "Exploitation," 156.

38. This case is described and modeled in Paul Seabright, "Blood, Bribes and the Crowding-Out of Altruism by Financial Incentives," unpublished manuscript, Université de Toulouse-1, February 2002.

39. Titmuss, *Gift Relationship,* 311.

40. Virginia Berridge, *AIDS in the UK: The Making of Policy, 1981–1994* (Oxford: Oxford University Press, 1996), 37–39; G. M. Gaul, "America: OPEC of Global Plasma Industry," *Philadelphia Inquirer,* September 28, 1989, A1.

41. Émile Durkheim, *The Division of Labor in Society* (New York: Free Press, 1984), 122.

42. Rene Almeling, "Gendering Commodification: How Egg Donation Agencies and Sperm Banks Structure Medical Markets in Genetic Material," master's thesis, University of California, Los Angeles, Sociology Department, 2003, p. 5.

43. George A. Akerlof, "Labor Contracts as Partial Gift Exchange," *Quarterly Journal of Economics* 97 (1982): 543–69.

44. Just as in Latin American politics Brazil is the country of the future—and always will be—so in transplant circles, the widespread application of xenotransplantation or artificial organs is always just a few years over the horizon.

45. See James Boyle, *Shamans, Software and Spleens: Law and the Construction of the Information Society* (Cambridge, MA: Harvard University Press, 1997).

46. Titmuss, *Gift Relationship,* 225.

47. Singer, "Altruism and Commerce," p. 319.

48. *Romeo and Juliet* 2.2.141–43.

49. Albert Hirschman, "Against Parsimony," in *Rival Views of Market Society* (Cambridge, MA: Harvard University Press, 1992) p. 157.

Bibliography

Akerlof, George A. "Labor Contracts as Partial Gift Exchange." *Quarterly Journal of Economics* 97 (1982): 543–69.

Alexander, G. C., and A. R. Seghal. "Barriers to Cadaveric Renal Transplantation among Blacks, Women, and the Poor." *Journal of the American Medical Association* 280, no. 13 (1998): 1148–52.

Alexander, Victoria. "Environmental Constraints and Organizational Strategies." In Powell and Clemens, *Private Action and the Public Good,* 272–90.

Allison, Paul. "The Cultural Evolution of Beneficial Norms." *Social Forces* 71 (1992): 279–301.

Almeling, Rene. "Gendering Commodification: How Egg Donation Agencies and Sperm Banks Structure Medical Markets in Genetic Material." Master's thesis, University of California, Los Angeles, Sociology Department, 2003.

Altman, L. K. "Use of Commercial Blood Increases with Shortages in U.S." *New York Times,* September 5, 1970, A1, A12.

Anderson, Elizabeth. *Value in Ethics and Economics.* Cambridge, MA: Harvard University Press, 1993.

Andrews, Lori, and Dorothy Nelkin. *Body Bazaar: The Market for Human Tissue in the Biotechnology Age.* New York: Crown, 2001.

Appadurai, Arjun. "Commodities and the Politics of Value." In *The Social Life of Things,* edited by Arjun Appadurai, 3–63. Cambridge: Cambridge University Press, 1986.

Arrow, Kenneth. "Gifts and Exchanges." *Philosophy and Public Affairs* 1, no. 4 (1972): 343–62.

Austin, W. "Sex Differences in Bystander Intervention in a Theft." *Journal of Personality and Social Psychology* 37 (1979): 2110–20.

Axelrod, Robert. *The Evolution of Cooperation.* New York: Basic Books, 1984.

Axelrod, Robert, and W. D. Hamilton. "The Evolution of Cooperation." *Science* 211 (1981): 1390–96.

Ayanian, J. Z., P. D. Cleary, J. S. Weissman, and A. M. Epstein. "The Effect of Patients' Preferences on Racial Differences in Access to Renal Transplantation." *New England Journal of Medicine* 341, no. 22 (1999): 1661–69.

Banevicius, Maria. "An Investigation of Cadaver Organ Donor Families Three Years after Donation: A Pilot Study." Master's thesis, Yale University School of Nursing, 1992.

Barman, Emily. "Asserting Difference: The Strategic Response of Nonprofit Organizations to Competition." *Social Forces* 80 (2002): 1191–1222.

Batson, C. D. "Prosocial Motivation: Is It Ever Truly Altruistic?" In *Advances in Experimental Social Psychology,* vol. 20, edited by L. Berkowitz, 65–122. New York: Academic Press, 1987.

Batten, Helen Levine, and Jeffrey Prottas. "Kind Strangers: The Families of Organ Donors." *Health Affairs* 6 (1987): 35–47.

Bauer, Stuart. "Blood Farming." *New York,* May 19, 1975, 50–70.

Bearman, Peter. *Doormen.* Chicago: University of Chicago Press, 2005.

———. "Generalized Exchange." *American Journal of Sociology* 102 (1997): 1383–1415.

Beck, Ulrich. *Risk Society.* London: Sage, 1992.

Beckert, Jens. "What Is Sociological about Economic Sociology? Uncertainty and the Embeddedness of Economic Action." *Theory and Society* 25 (1996): 803–40.

Bekkers, Rene. *Giving and Volunteering in the Netherlands: Sociological and Psychological Perspectives.* Amsterdam: Thesis Publishers (Utrecht University), 2004.

Bender, Courtney. *Heaven's Kitchen: Living Religion at God's Love We Deliver.* Chicago: University of Chicago Press, 2003.

Berridge, Virginia. *AIDS in the UK: The Making of Policy, 1981–1994.* Oxford: Oxford University Press, 1996.

Blair, Roger, and David Kaserman. "The Economics and Ethics of Alternative Cadaveric Organ Procurement Policies." *Yale Journal of Regulation* 8 (1991): 403–52.

Bosk, Charles L. "Professional Ethicist Available: Logical, Secular, Friendly." *Dædalus* 128, no. 4 (1999): 47–68.

Bourdieu, Pierre. *Practical Reason.* Stanford: Stanford University Press, 1998.

Boyd, Robert, and Peter J. Richerson. *Culture and the Evolutionary Process.* Chicago: University of Chicago Press, 1985.

Boyle, James. *Shamans, Software and Spleens: Law and the Construction of the Information Society.* Cambridge, MA: Harvard University Press, 1997.

Bradley, M. B., Norman M. Green Jr., Dale E. Jones, Mac Lynn, and Lou McNeil. "Churches and Church Membership in the United States." Washington, DC: Glenmary Research Center, 1992.

Callon, Michel, ed. *The Laws of the Market.* Oxford: Blackwell, 1998.

Caplan, Arthur. *If I Were a Rich Man, Could I Buy a Pancreas?* Indiana: Indiana University Press, 1994.

———. "Sounding Board: Ethical and Policy Issues in the Procurement of Cadaver Organs for Transplantation." *New England Journal of Medicine* 311 (1984): 981–83.

Caplan, Arthur, and Daniel Coelho, eds. *The Ethics of Organ Transplants.* Amherst: Prometheus Books, 1998.

Caplow, Theodore. "Christmas Gifts and Kin Networks." *American Sociological Review* 47 (1982): 383–92.

Caputo, Phillip. "Blood Banks: Pay Stations." *Chicago Tribune,* September 14, 1971.

Carney, Karen. *Precious Gifts: Katie Coolican's Story. Barklay and Eve Explain Organ and Tissue Donation.* N.p.: Dragonfly Publishing, 1999.

Carrier, James. "Gifts, Commodities and Social Relations: A Maussian View of Exchange." *Sociological Forum* 6 (1991): 119–36.

Carruthers, Bruce, and Arthur Stinchcombe. "The Social Structure of Liquidity: Flexibility, Markets and States." *Theory and Society* 28 (1999): 353–82.

Chang, Ruth. *Incommensurability, Incomparability and Practical Reason.* Cambridge, MA: Harvard University Press, 1997.

Chaves, Mark. "The Religious Ethic and the Spirit of Nonprofit Entrepreneurship." In Powell and Clemens, *Private Action and the Public Good,* 47–68.

Childress, James F. "Ethical Criteria for Procuring and Distributing Organs for Transplantation." *Journal of Health Politics, Policy and Law* 14 (1989): 87–113.

Christiansen, C. L., S. L. Gortmaker, J. M. Williams, C. L. Beasley, L. E. Brigham, C. Capossela, M. E. Matthiesen, and S. Gunderson. "A Method for Estimating Solid Organ Donor Potential by Organ Procurement Region." *American Journal of Public Health* 88, no. 11 (1998): 1645–50.

Churchill, Larry R., and Rosa Lynn Pinkus. "The Use of Anencephalic Organs: Historical and Ethical Dimensions." *Milbank Quarterly* 68 (1990): 147–69.

Clarke, Lee, and Carroll Estes. "Sociological and Economic Theories of Markets and Nonprofits: Evidence from Home Health Organizations." *American Journal of Sociology* 97 (1992): 945–69.

Clarke, Lee, and James F. Short. "Social Organization and Risk: Some Current Controversies." *Annual Review of Sociology* 19 (1993): 375–99.

Clotfelter, C. "On Trends in Private Sources of Support for the US Non-profit Sector." *Voluntas* 4, no. 2 (1993): 190–95.

Cohen, G. A. *Karl Marx's Theory of History: A Defence.* Expanded ed. Princeton: Princeton University Press, 2000.

Cohen, Lawrence. "Where It Hurts: Indian Material for an Ethics of Organ Transplantation." *Dædalus* 128, no. 4 (1999): 135–66.

Cohen, Lloyd. "Increasing the Supply of Transplant Organs: The Virtues of a Futures Market." *George Washington Law Review* 58 (1989): 1–51.

Committee to Study HIV Transmission through Blood Products. "Proceedings of a Public Meeting Held on September 12, 1994, in Washington D.C." (Department of Commerce, 1994). National Technical Information Service record locator number PB95-142345.

Cooper, David K., and Robert P. Lanza. *Xeno: The Promise of Transplanting Animal Organs into Humans.* New York: Oxford University Press, 2000.

Culyer, A. J. "Blood and Altruism: An Economic Review." In Johnson, *Blood Policy,* 29–58.

Dennis, Michael J. "Scarce Medical Resources: Hemodialysis and Kidney Transplantation." In *Local Justice in America,* edited by Jon Elster, 81–152. New York: Russell Sage Foundation, 1995.

Dossick, Phillip. *Transplant: A Family Chronicle.* New York: Viking, 1978.

Douglas, Mary. *Risk and Blame.* New York: Routledge, 1982.

Drake, A. W., S. N. Finkelstein, and H. M. Sapolsky. *The American Blood Supply.* Cambridge, MA: MIT Press, 1982.

Durkheim, Emile. *The Division of Labor in Society.* Translated by W. D. Halls. New York: Free Press, 1984.

Dutton, Diana. *Worse Than the Disease.* New York: Cambridge University Press, 1988.

Economist. "The Return of the Bodysnatchers." February 3, 2001, 59–60.

Edds, Kimberly. "UCLA Denies Role in Cadaver Case." *Washington Post,* March 9, 2004, A03.

Ehrle, R. N., T. J. Shafer, and K. R. Nelson. "Referral, Request and Consent for Organ Donation: Best Practice—A Blueprint for Success." *Critical Care Nurse* 19 (1999): 21–33.

Ekeh, Peter. *Social Exchange Theory: The Two Traditions.* Cambridge, MA: Harvard University Press, 1974.

Elster, Jon. "Selfishness and Altruism." In *Beyond Self-Interest,* edited by Jane J. Mansbridge, 44–53. Chicago: University of Chicago Press, 1990.

———. *Sour Grapes.* New York: Cambridge University Press, 1983.

———. *Ulysses and the Sirens.* New York: Cambridge University Press, 1984.

Espeland, Wendy Nelson, and Mitchell L. Stevens. "Commensuration as a Social Process." *Annual Review of Sociology* 24 (1998): 313–43.

Etzioni, Amitai. *The Moral Dimension: Toward a New Economics.* New York: Free Press, 1988.

Evans, John H. *Playing God? Human Genetic Engineering and the Rationalization of Bioethics, 1959–1995.* Chicago: University of Chicago Press, 2001.

Evans, R., C. Orians, and N. Ascher. "The Potential Supply of Organ Donors." *Journal of the American Medical Association* 267, no. 2 (1992): 239–46.

Feldman, Eric A., and Ronald Bayer, eds. *Blood Feuds: AIDS, Blood, and the Politics of Medical Disaster.* New York: Oxford University Press, 1999.

Feldman, Martha S., and James G. March. "Information in Organizations as Signal and Symbol." *Administrative Science Quarterly* 26 (1981): 171–86.

Finlay, T. *Report of the Tribunal of Inquiry into the Blood Transfusion Service Board.* Dublin: Stationery Office, 1997.

Finucane, M., P. Slovic, and C. Mertz. "Public Perception of the Risk of Blood Transfusion." *Transfusion* 40 (2000): 1017–22.

Fox, Renée, and Judith Swazey. *The Courage to Fail: A Social View of Organ Transplantation and Dialysis.* Chicago: University of Chicago Press, 1974.

———. *Spare Parts: Organ Replacement in American Society.* New York: Oxford University Press, 1992.

Frank, Robert, Thomas Gilovich, and Dennis Regan. "Does Studying Economics Inhibit Cooperation?" *Journal of Economic Perspectives* 7 (1993): 159–72.

Frey, Bruno. "A Constitution for Knaves Crowds out Civic Virtues." *Economic Journal* 107 (1997): 1043–53.

Frey, B. S., F. OberholzerGee, and R. Eichenberger. "The Old Lady Visits Your Backyard: A Tale of Morals and Markets." *Journal of Political Economy* 104, no. 6 (1996): 1297–1313.

Friedland, Roger, and Robert R. Alford. "Bringing Society Back In: Symbols, Practices and Institutional Contradictions." In *The New Institutionalism and Organizational Analysis,* edited by Walter Powell and Paul DiMaggio, 232–66. Chicago: University of Chicago Press, 1991.

Frumkin, Peter. *On Being Nonprofit: A Conceptual and Policy Primer.* Cambridge, MA: Harvard University Press, 2002.

Gallup Organization. "The American Public's Attitudes toward Organ Donation and Transplantation: A Survey Conducted for the Partnership for Organ Donation." Boston, February 1993.

Gaul, G. M. "America: OPEC of Global Plasma Industry." *Philadelphia Inquirer,* September 28, 1989, A1.

General Accounting Office. *Organ Procurement Organizations: Alternatives Being Developed to More Accurately Assess Performance.* Washington, DC: General Accounting Office, 1997. GAO/HEHS-98-26.

———. *Organ Transplants: Increased Effort Needed to Boost Supply and Ensure Equitable Distribution of Organs.* Washington, DC: General Accounting Office, 1993. GAO/HRD-93-56.

Genetet, Bernard. *Blood Transfusion: Half a Century of Contribution by the Council of Europe.* Strasbourg: Council of Europe, 1998.

Godelier, Maurice. *The Enigma of the Gift.* Chicago: University of Chicago Press, 1999.

Goffman, Erving. "On Cooling the Mark Out: Some Aspects of Adaptation to Failure." *Psychiatry* 15 (1952): 451–63.

Gortmaker, Steven L. "Improving the Request Process to Increase Family Consent for Organ Donation." *Journal of Transplant Coordination* 8 (1998): 210–17.

———. "Organ Donor Potential and Performance: Size and Nature of the Organ Donor Shortfall." *Critical Care Medicine* 24 (1996): 432–39.

Granovetter, Mark. "Economic Action and Social Structure: The Problem of Embeddedness." *American Journal of Sociology* 91 (1985): 481–510.

Greeley, Andrew. "The Other Civic America: Religion and Social Capital." *American Prospect* 32 (1997): 68–73.

Green, Reg, *The Nicholas Effect: A Boy's Gift to the World.* Sebastopol, CA: O'Reilly, 1999.

Gregory, C. A. *Gifts and Commodities.* London: Academic Press, 1982.

———. "Gifts to Men and Gifts to God: Gift Exchange and Capital Accumulation in Contemporary Papua." *Man* 15 (1980): 626–52.

Grønbjerg, Kirsten. *Understanding Nonprofit Funding: Managing Revenues in Social Service and Community Development Organizations.* (San Francisco: Jossey-Bass, 1993.

Guadagnoli, E., P. McNamara, M. J. Evanisko, C. Beasley, C. O. Callender, and A. Poretsky. "The Influence of Race on Approaching Families for Organ Donation and Their Decision to Donate." *American Journal of Public Health* 89, no. 2 (1999): 244–47.

Gutkind, Lee. *Many Sleepless Nights: The World of Organ Transplantation.* (Pittsburgh: University of Pittsburgh Press, 1990.

Hagen, Piet. *Blood Transfusion in Europe: A White Paper.* Strasbourg: Council of Europe, 1993.

Hamilton, W. D. "The Genetical Evolution of Social Behavior." Pts. 1 and 2. *Journal of Theoretical Biology* 7 (1964): 1–16, 17–52.

Hansmann, Henry. "The Economics and Ethics of Markets for Human Organs." *Journal of Health Politics, Policy and Law* 14 (1989): 57–85.

Harrell, Frank E. *Regression Modeling Strategies.* New York: Springer, 2001.

Hausman, Daniel M., and Michael S. McPherson. *Economic Analysis and Moral Philosophy.* New York: Cambridge University Press, 1996.

Hedges, Stephen J., and William Gaines. "Donor Bodies Milled into Growing Profits." *Chicago Tribune,* May 21, 2000, A1, A16–17.

Heimer, Carol. "Allocating Information Costs in a Negotiated Information Order: Interorganizational Constraints on Decision Making in Norwegian Oil Insurance." *Administrative Science Quarterly* 30 (1985): 395–417.

———. "Social Structure, Psychology and the Estimation of Risk." *Annual Review of Sociology* 14 (1988): 491–519.

Heisel, William, and Mark Katches. "Organ Agencies Aid For-Profit Suppliers." *Orange County Register,* June 25, 2000, http://www.ocregister.com/features/body/organ00625cci.shtml.

Henrich, Joseph, Robert Boyd, Samuel Bowles, Colin Camerer, Ernst Fehr, Herbert Gintis, and Richard McElreath. "In Search of Homo Economicus: Behavioral Experiments in 15 Small-Scale Societies." *American Economic Review* 91 (2001): 73–78.

Hirschman, Albert. "Against Parsimony." In *Rival Views of Market Society,* 142–60. Cambridge, MA: Harvard University Press, 1992.

———. *The Passions and the Interests.* Princeton: Princeton University Press, 1978.

Hochschild, Arlie Russell. *The Commercialization of Intimate Life.* Berkeley: University of California Press, 2003.

———. *The Managed Heart: Commercialization of Human Feeling.* Berkeley: University of California Press, 1985.

Hodgkinson, V., and M. Weitzman. *Giving and Volunteering in the United States: Findings from a National Survey.* Washington, DC: Independent Sector, 1992.

Hoffman, M. L. "Is Altruism Part of Human Nature?" *Journal of Personality and Social Psychology* 40 (1981): 121–37.

Hogle, Linda. *Recovering the Nation's Body: Cultural Memory, Medicine and the Politics of Redemption.* New Brunswick, NJ: Rutgers University Press, 1999.

Horton, Raymond L., and Patricia J. Horton. "Knowledge Regarding Organ Dona-
    tion: Identifying and Overcoming Barriers to Organ Donation." *Social Science
    and Medicine* 31 (1990): 791–800.
Institute of Medicine. *HIV and the Blood Supply: An Analysis of Crisis Decision-
    making.* Washington, DC: National Academy Press, 1995.
———. *Organ Procurement and Transplantation.* Washington, DC: National Acad-
    emy Press, 1999.
Jencks, Christopher. "Who Gives to What?" In *The Nonprofit Sector: A Research
    Handbook,* edited by Walter W. Powell, 331–39. New Haven: Yale University
    Press, 1992.
Jendrisak, M. D., K. Hruska, J. Wagner, D. Chandler, and D. Kappel. "Cadaveric-
    Donor Organ Recovery at a Hospital-Independent Facility." *Transplantation*
    74, no. 7 (2002): 931–32.
Jewish Voice, "Organ Transplant: Soon It May Be a Routine Part of the Jewish Death
    Ritual," December 1996.
Johnson, David B., ed. *Blood Policy: Issues and Alternatives.* Washington, DC: Ameri-
    can Enterprise Institute for Public Policy Research, 1976.
Kaserman, David, and A. H. Barnett. *The U.S. Organ Procurement System: A Prescrip-
    tion for Reform.* Washington, DC: American Enterprise Institute Press, 2002.
Kasiske, B.L., J. F. Neylan, R. R. Riggio, G. M. Danovtich, L. Kahana, S. R. Alexan-
    der, and M. G. White. "The Effect of Race on Access and Outcome in Trans-
    plantation." *New England Journal of Medicine* 324 (1991): 320–27.
Katches, Mark, and William Heisel. "Preliminary Tissue-Trade Report Issued."
    Orange County Register, August 9, 2000, http://www.ocregister.com/features/
    body/body00809.shtml.
Kelly, David, and Walter Wiest. "Christian Perspectives." In Keyes and Wiest, *New
    Harvest,* 199–221.
Kessel, Reuben. "Transfused Blood, Serum Hepatitis and the Coase Theorem."
    In Johnson, *Blood Policy,* 183–207.
Keyes, C. Don, and Walter E. Wiest, eds. *New Harvest: Transplanting the Body and
    Reaping the Benefits.* Clifton, NJ: Humana Press, 1991.
Kimbrell, Andrew. *The Human Body Shop: The Cloning, Engineering and Marketing of
    Life.* 2nd ed. Washington, DC: Regnery, 1998.
Klassen, Ann C., and David K. Klassen. "Who Are the Donors in Organ Donation?
    The Family's Perspective in Mandated Choice." *Annals of Internal Medicine*
    125 (1996): 70–73.
Klassen, A. C., D. K. Klassen, R. Aronoff, A. G. Hall, and J. Braslow. "Organiza-
    tional Characteristics of Solid-Organ Donor Hospitals and Nondonor Hospi-
    tals." *Journal of Transplant Coordination* 9 (1999): 87–94.
Kopfman, J. E., S. W. Smith, K. Morrison, and H. J. Yoo. "Influence of Race on Cog-
    nitive and Affective Reactions to Organ Donation Messages." *Transplantation
    Proceedings* 34 (2002): 3035–41.
Krebs, D. K., and D. T. Miller. "Altruism and Aggression." In *Handbook of Social
    Psychology,* 3rd ed. edited by G. Lindzey and E. Aronson, 2:1–71. New York:
    Random House, 1985.

Lamb, David. *Organ Transplants and Ethics.* New York: Routledge, 1990.

Landes, Elizabeth, and Richard Posner. "The Economics of the Baby Shortage." *Journal of Legal Studies* 7 (1978): 323–48.

Latané, B., and J. M. Darley. "Social Determinants of Bystander Intervention in Emergencies." In *Altruism and Helping Behavior: Social Psychological Studies of Some Antecedents and Consequences,* edited by J. Macaulay and L. Berkowitz, 13–27. New York: Academic Press, 1970.

Lee, Lichang, Jane Allyn Piliavin, and Vaughn R. A. Call. "Giving Time, Money and Blood: Similarities and Differences." *Social Psychology Quarterly* 62 (1999): 276–90.

Lindblom, Charles E. *The Market System.* New Haven: Yale University Press, 2002.

Lock, Margaret. "Deadly Disputes: Ideologies and Brain Death in Japan." In Younger, Fox, and O'Connell, *Organ Transplantation,* 142–67.

———. *Twice Dead: Organ Transplants and the Reinvention of Death.* Berkeley: University of California Press, 2002.

London, P., and B. M. Hemphill. "The Motivations of Blood Donors." *Transfusion* 14 (1965): 559–68.

Macy, Michael, and John Skvoretz. "The Evolution of Trust and Cooperation Between Strangers: A Computational Model." *American Sociological Review* 63 (1998): 638–60.

Madigan, Nick. "Inquiry Widens after 2 Arrests in Cadaver Case at UCLA." *New York Times,* March 9, 2004, A21.

Malinowski, Bronislaw. *Argonauts of the Western Pacific.* London: Routledge, 1922.

———. *Crime and Custom in Savage Society.* London: Routledge, 1926.

Mark, Noah. "The Cultural Evolution of Cooperation." *American Sociological Review* 67, no. 3 (2002): 323–44.

Marwell, Gerald, and Ruth Ames. "Economists Free Ride: Does Anyone Else?" *Journal of Public Economics* 15 (1981): 295–310.

Marx, Karl. *Capital.* Vol. 1. Translated by Ben Fowkes. London: Penguin, 1990.

———. "Inaugural Address of the International Working Men's Association." In *The Marx-Engels Reader,* 2nd ed., edited by Robert C. Tucker, 512–19. New York: Norton, 1978.

———. "On James Mill." In *Karl Marx: Selected Writings,* edited by David McLellan, 124–33. London: Oxford University Press, 2000.

———. "Wage-Labour and Capital." In *Karl Marx: Selected Writings,* edited by David McLellan, 273–94. London: Oxford University Press, 2000.

Mauss, Marcel. *The Gift: The Form and Reason for Exchange in Archaic Societies.* New York: Norton, 2000.

Mead, Rebecca. "Eggs for Sale." *New Yorker,* August 9, 1999, 56–65.

Miller, Dale. "The Norm of Self Interest." *American Psychologist* 54, no. 12 (1999): 1–8.

Miller, Dale T., and Rebecca Ratner. "The Power of the Myth of Self-Interest." In *Current Societal Issues In Justice,* edited by L. Montada and M. Lerner, 25–48. New York: Plenum Press, 1996.

Monroe, Kristen Renwick. *The Heart of Altruism.* Princeton: Princeton University Press, 1998.

Nathan, H. M. "Pennsylvania Looks for Answers to the Organ Donor Shortage." Press release. Gift of Life Donor Program, Pittsburgh, June 10, 1999.

National Research Council archive of background material provided to the Institute of Medicine's Committee to Study HIV Transmission through Blood and Blood Products. Transcript of Blood Products Advisory Council meeting, December 4, 1982.

———.Transcript of Blood Products Advisory Council meeting, February 7–8, 1983. Box 3, tab 86.

———. Joseph Bove interview notes, 1994. Box 2, folder 25.

———. Bruce Evatt interview notes, 1983. Box 2, folder 25.

———. Minutes of National Hemophilia Foundation meeting, October 22, 1983. Box 3.

———. June Osborn interview notes, 1994. Box 2, folder 25.

Nelson, Julie. "One Sphere or Two?" *American Behavioral Scientist* 41, no. 10 (1998): 1467–71.

New York Times. "Pope Warns of Danger in Organ Transplants and Genetic Testing." October 27, 1980, A1.

Norris, M. K. Gaedeke. "Required Request: Why It Has Not Significantly Improved the Donor Shortage." *Heart & Lung* 19 (1990): 685–86.

Nussbaum, Martha. "'Whether from Reason or Prejudice': Taking Money for Bodily Services." *Journal of Legal Studies* 27 (June 1998): 693–724.

O'Carroll, J. P. "Blood." In *Encounters with Modern Ireland,* edited by M. Peillon and E. Slater, 107–14. Dublin: Institute of Public Administration, 1999.

Office of Evaluation and Inspections. *Oversight of Tissue Banking.* Washington, DC: Department of Health and Human Services, 2001. OEI 01-00-00441.

Oliner, S. P., and P. M. Oliner. *The Altruistic Personality: Rescuers of Jews in Nazi Europe.* New York: Free Press, 1988.

Oliver, Christine. "Strategic Responses to Institutional Processes." *Academy of Management Review* 16 (1991): 145–79.

O'Neill, Onora. *Autonomy and Trust in Bioethics.* Cambridge: Cambridge University Press, 2002.

Oswalt, R. M. "A Review of Blood Donor Motivation and Recruitment." *Transfusion* 17 (1977): 123–35.

Oswalt, R. M., and T. E. Hoff. "The Motivations of Blood Donors and Non-donors: A Community Survey," *Transfusion* 15 (1975): 68–72.

Ozcan, Y. A., J. W. Begun, and M. M. McKinney. "Benchmarking Organ Procurement Organizations: A National Study." *Health Services Research* 34, no. 4 (1999): 855–74.

Panem, Sandra. *The AIDS Bureaucracy.* Cambridge, MA: Harvard University Press, 1998.

Parr, Elizabeth. *I'm Glad You're Not Dead: A Liver Transplant Story.* New York: Journey, 1996.

Parry, Jonathan. "The Gift, the Indian Gift and the'Indian Gift.'" *Man* 21 (1986): 453–73.

Parry, Jonathan, and Maurice Bloch, eds. *Money and the Morality of Exchange*. Cambridge: Cambridge University Press, 1989.

Pekkanen, John. *Donor: How One Girl's Death Gave Life to Others*. Boston: Little, Brown, 1986.

Perlmutter, Ted. "Italy: Why No Voluntary Sector?" In *Between States and Markets: The Voluntary Sector in Comparative Perspective,* edited by Robert Wuthnow, 157–88. Princeton: Princeton University Press, 1991.

Perrow, Charles, and Mauro F. Guillen. *The AIDS Disaster*. New Haven: Yale University Press, 1990.

Pfeffer, Jeffrey, and Gerald Salancik. *The External Dependence of Organizations: A Resource Dependence Perspective*. New York: Harper and Row, 1978.

Piliavin, J. A. "Why Do They Give the Gift of Life? A Review of Research on Blood Donors since 1977." *Transfusion* 30 (1990): 444–59.

Piliavin, Jane Allyn, and Peter L. Callero. *Giving Blood: The Development of an Altruistic Identity*. Baltimore: Johns Hopkins University Press, 1991.

Piliavin, Jane Allyn, and Hong-Wen Charng. "Altruism: A Review of Recent Theory and Research." *Annual Review of Sociology* 16 (1990): 27–65.

Polanyi, Karl. *The Great Transformation: The Political and Economic Origins of Our Time*. Boston: Beacon Press, 1980.

Poole, Victoria. *Thursday's Child*. New York: Little, Brown, 1980.

Powell, Walter W., and Elisabeth S. Clemens, eds. *Private Action and the Public Good*. New Haven: Yale University Press, 1998.

Powner, David J., and Joseph M. Darby. "Current Considerations in the Issue of Brain Death." *Neurosurgery* 45 (1999): 1222–27.

Prottas, Jeffrey. *The Most Useful Gift: Altruism and the Public Policy of Organ Transplants*. San Francisco: Jossey Bass, 1994.

———. "The Organization of Organ Procurement." *Journal of Health Politics, Policy and Law* 14, no. 1 (1989): 41–55.

Putnam, Robert. *Bowling Alone: The Collapse and Revival of American Community*. New York: Simon and Schuster, 2000.

R Core Development Team. "R: A Language and Environment for Statistical Computing." Vienna: R Foundation for Statistical Computing, 2003. http://www.r-project.org.

Rabin, Matthew. "Psychology and Economics." *Journal of Economic Literature* 36 (1998): 11–46.

Rabinow, Paul. *French DNA: Trouble in Purgatory*. Chicago: University of Chicago Press, 1999.

Radin, Margaret. *Contested Commodities*. Cambridge, MA: Harvard University Press, 1996.

Randall, V. R. "Slavery, Segregation and Racism: Trusting the Medical System Ain't Always Easy! An African-American Perspective on Bioethics." *St. Louis University Public Law Review* 15 (1996): 181–235.

Redfern, Michael. *The Royal Liverpool Children's Inquiry.* Liverpool: United Kingdom Department of Health, 2001.

Reif, Karlheinz, and Eric Marlier. *Eurobarometer 41.0.* Machine-readable data file. Ann Arbor: Inter-University Consortium for Political Research, 1995.

Ribal, Lizzy. *Lizzy Gets a New Liver.* Louisville, KY: Bridge Resources, 1997.

Richardson, Ruth. "Fearful Symmetry: Corpses for Anatomy, Organs for Transplant?" In Younger, Fox, and O'Connell, *Organ Transplantation,* 66–100.

Rifkin, Jeremy. *The Biotech Century.* New York: Tarcher, 1999.

Roberts, R. D., and M. D. Wolkoff. "Improving the Quality of Whole-Blood Supply: Limits to Voluntary Arrangements." *Journal of Health Policy, Politics and Law* 13 (1988): 167–78.

Royle, Nicholas. *The Matter of the Heart.* London: Abacus, 1997.

Rozon-Solomon, M., and L. Burrows. "'Tis Better to Receive Than to Give: The Relative Failure of the African American Community to Provide Organs for Transplantation." *Mount Sinai Journal of Medicine* 66, no. 4 (1999): 273–76.

Sade, Robert M., Nancy Kay, Steve Pitzer, Peggy Drake, Prabhakar Baliga, and Stephen Haines. "Increasing Organ Donation: A Successful New Concept." *Transplantation* 72 (2002): 1142–46.

Sahlins, Marshall. *Stone Age Economics.* Chicago: Aldine, 1972.

Salamon, Lester M., and Anheier, Helmut K. *The Nonprofit Sector in Comparative Perspective: An Overview.* Baltimore: Johns Hopkins University Press, 1994.

Sammons, Bonnie Harris. "Organ Recovery Coordinators Can Help Family Work through the Grieving Process." *AORN Journal* 48 (1988): 181–82.

Sapolsky, H. M., and S. L. Boswell. "The History of Transfusion AIDS: Practice and Policy Alternatives." In *AIDS: The Making of a Chronic Disease,* edited by Elizabeth Fee and Daniel M. Fox, 170–93. Berkeley: University of California Press, 1992.

Sapolsky, H. M., and S. N. Finkelstein. "Blood Policy Revisited—A New Look at the Gift Relationship." *Public Interest* 46 (1977): 15–27.

Scheper-Hughes, Nancy. "The Global Traffic in Human Organs." *Current Anthropology* 41, no. 2 (2000): 191–211.

———. *Parts Unknown: The Global Traffic in Human Organs.* New York: Farrar, Strauss and Giroux, forthcoming.

Scheper-Hughes, Nancy, and Loïc Waquant, eds. *Commodifying Bodies.* Thousand Oaks, CA: Sage, 2002.

Schervish, Paul G., and John J. Havens. "Social Participation and Charitable Giving: A Multivariate Analysis." *Voluntas* 8 (1997): 235–60.

Schlesinger, Mark. "Mismeasuring the Consequences of Ownership: External Influences and the Comparative Performance of Public, For-Profit, and Private Nonprofit Organizations." In Powell and Clemens, *Private Action and the Public Good,* 85–113.

Schmidt, P. "Blood and Disaster: Supply and Demand." *New England Journal of Medicine* 346 (2002): 617–20.

Schmidtz, David. "Reasons for Altruism." *Social Philosophy and Policy* 10, no. 1 (1993): 52–68.

Schofer, Evan, and Marion Fourcade-Gourinchas. "The Structural Contexts of Civic Engagement: Voluntary Association Membership in Comparative Perspectice." *American Sociological Review* 66 (2001): 806–28.

Schomaker, Mary Zimmeth. *Lifeline: How One Night Changed Five Lives.* New York: New Horizon Press, 1995.

Scott, Marvin B., and Stanford M. Lyman. "Accounts." *American Sociological Review* 33, no. 1 (1968): 46–62.

Seabright, Paul. "Blood, Bribes and the Crowding-Out of Altruism by Financial Incentives." Unpublished manuscript, Université de Toulouse-1, February 2002.

Shafer, T. J. "Two Years Experience with Routine Notification." Paper presented at the annual meeting of the North American Transplant Coordinators Organization, New York, August 10, 1998.

Shanteau, J., and R. Harris, eds. *Organ Donation and Transplantation: Psychological and Behavioral Factors.* Washington, DC: APA Press, 1990.

Shilts, Randy. *And the Band Played On: Politics, People and the AIDS Epidemic.* New York: St. Martin's Press, 1988.

Siegel, Reva B. "The Modernization of Marital Status Law: Adjudicating Wives' Rights to Earnings, 1860–1930." *Georgetown Law Journal* 82 (September 1994): 2127–2211.

Silbaugh, Katharine. "Turning Labor into Love: Housework and the Law." *Northwestern University Law Review* 91 (1996): 1–85.

Silver, Allan. "Friendship in Commercial Society: Eighteenth-Century Social Theory and Modern Sociology." *American Journal of Sociology* 95, no. 6 (1990): 1474–1504.

Siminoff, Laura, Nahida Gordon, Joan Hewlett, and Robert Arnold. "Factors Influencing Families' Consent for Donation of Solid Organs for Transplantation." *Journal of the American Medical Association* 286, no. 1 (July 4, 2001): 71–77.

Siminoff, Laura, and Kristine Nelson. "The Accuracy of Hospital Reports of Organ Donation Eligibility, Requests and Consent: A Cross-Validation Study." *Joint Commission Journal on Quality Improvement* 25, no. 3 (1999): 129–36.

Simmons, Roberta G. "Altruism and Sociology." *Sociological Quarterly* 32 (1991): 1–22.

Simmons, Roberta, Susan Klein Marine, and Richard Simmons. *Gift of Life: The Social and Psychological Impact of Organ Transplantation.* New York: Wiley, 1977.

Singer, Peter. "Altruism and Commerce: A Defense of Titmuss against Arrow." *Philosophy and Public Affairs* 2, no. 3 (1973): 312–20.

Skocpol, Theda, Marshal Ganz, and Ziah Munson. "A Nation of Organizers: The Institutional Origins of Civic Voluntarism in the United States." *American Political Science Review* 94 (2000): 527–46.

Smith, John Maynard. *Evolution and the Theory of Games.* New York: Cambridge University Press, 1982.

———. "Group Selection and Kin Selection." *Nature* 201 (1964): 1145–46.

Snowbeck, Christoper. "Organ Donor Funeral Aid Scrapped." *Pittsburgh Post Gazette,* February 1, 2002, B1.

Sober, Elliot, and David Sloan Wilson. *Unto Others: The Evolution and Psychology of Unselfish Behavior.* Cambridge, MA: Harvard University Press, 1998.

Southeastern Institute of Research. "General Consumers: American Attitudes toward the Allocation of Organ Transplantation." Richmond, VA: United Network for Organ Sharing, 1994.

Spray, Glenys. *Blood, Sweat and Tears: The Hepatitis C Scandal.* Dublin: Wolfhound Press, 1998.

Starr, Douglas. *Blood: An Epic History of Medicine and Commerce.* New York: Knopf, 1998.

Starzl, Thomas. *The Puzzle People: Memoirs of a Transplant Surgeon.* Pittsburgh: University of Pittsburgh Press, 1992.

Stolberg, Sheryl Gay. "Pennsylvania Set to Break Taboo on Reward for Organ Donations." *New York Times,* May 6, 1999, A1.

Strange, Julie Mull, and David Taylor. "Organ and Tissue donation." In *Transplantation Nursing: Acute and Long-Term Management,* edited by Marie T. Nolan and Sharon M. Augustine, 77–108. Norwalk: Appleton & Lange, 1991.

Strom, Stephanie. "Extreme Philanthropy: Giving of Yourself, Literally, to People You've Never Met." *New York Times,* July 27, 2003, D3.

———. "An Organ Donor's Generosity Raises the Question of How Much Is Too Much?" *New York Times,* August 17, 2003, A14.

Sunstein, Cass. *Free Markets and Social Justice.* New York: Oxford University Press, 1997.

———. "Incommensurability and Kinds of Valuation." In Chang, *Incommensurability, Incomparability and Practical Reason,* 234–54.

Sylvia, Claire. *A Change of Heart: A Memoir.* New York: Little, Brown, 1997.

Tilly, Charles. "Power—Top Down and Bottom Up." *Journal of Political Philosophy* 7 (1999): 330–52.

Titmuss, Richard. *The Gift Relationship: From Human Blood to Social Policy.* New York: Vintage, 1971.

———. *The Gift Relationship: From Human Blood to Social Policy.* Expanded and updated ed. New York: New Press, 1997.

Trivers, R. L. "The Evolution of Reciprocal Altruism." *Quarterly Review of Biology* 46 (1971): 35–57.

Twersky, Abraham, Michael Gold, and Walter Jacob. "Jewish Perspectives." In Keyes and Wiest, *New Harvest,* 187–98.

Ubel, Peter. *Pricing Life.* Cambridge, MA: MIT Press, 2000.

Ubel, Peter, Cindy Bryce, Laura Siminoff, Arthur Caplan, and Robert Arnold. "Pennsylvania's Voluntary Benefits Program: Evaluating an Innovative Proposal for Increasing Organ Donation." *Health Affairs* 19, no. 5 (2000): 206–11.

Ubel, Peter, and Arthur Caplan. "Geographic Favoritism in Liver Transplanta-tion—Unfortunate or Unfair?" *New England Journal of Medicine* 339, no. 18 (1998): 1322–25.

United Kingdom Department of Health. *Report of a Census of Organs and Tissues Retained by Pathology Services in England.* London, 2000.

United Network for Organ Sharing. *Donation & Transplantation: Nursing Curricu-lum.* Richmond, VA: UNOS, n.d.

———. *Organ and Tissue Donation: A Reference Guide for Clergy.* 3rd ed. Richmond, VA: UNOS, 1998.

———. "Share Your Life. Share Your Decision." Informational brochure, 1999.

———. *UNOS Organ Procurement Coordinator's Handbook.* Richmond, VA: UNOS, 1995.

Van Aken, W. G. *The Collection and Use of Human Blood and Plasma in Europe.* Strasbourg: Council of Europe Press, 1993.

Veith, Frank. "Organ Transplants and the Pope's Statement." Letter to the editor. *New York Times,* November 10, 1980, A22.

Venables, W. N., and B. D. Ripley. *Modern Applied Statistics with S.* 4th ed. New York: Springer, 2002.

Verble, Margaret, Gordon R. Bowen, Nancy Kay, Jeffrey Mitoff, Teresa J. Shafer, and Judy Worth. "A Multiethnic Study of the Relationship between Fears and Concerns and Refusal Rates." *Progress in Transplantation* 12, no. 3 (2002): 185–90.

Verble, Margaret, and Judy Worth. "Overcoming Families' Fears and Concerns in the Donation Discussion." *Progress in Transplantation* 10, no. 3 (2000): 155–60.

Waldby, Catherine, Marsha Rosengarten, Carla Treolar, and Suzanne Fraser. "Blood and Bioidentity: Ideas about Self, Boundaries and Risk among Blood Donors and People Living with Hepatitis C." *Social Science and Medicine* 59 (2004): 1461–71.

Walzer, Michael. *Spheres of Justice.* New York: Basic Books, 1983.

Weiner, Annette. *Inalienable Possessions: The Paradox of Keeping-while-Giving.* Berkeley: University of California Press, 1992.

Wendler, Dave, and Neal Dickert. "The Consent Process for Cadaveric Organ Pro-curement: How Does It Work? How Can It Be Improved?" *Journal of the Ameri-can Medical Association* 285, no. 3 (2001): 329–33.

Westfall, Pamela. "Hepatitis, AIDS and the Blood Products Exemption from Strict Products Liability in California: A Reassessment." *Hastings Law Journal* 37 (1986): 1101–32.

Williams, Barbara A. Helene, Kathleen L. Grady, and Doris M. Sadiford-Guttenbeil. *Organ Transplantation: A Manual for Nurses.* New York: Springer, 1991.

Williams, Joan. *Unbending Gender: Why Family and Work Conflict and What to Do about It.* New York: Oxford University Press, 1999.

Wolfe, Alan. "What Is Altruism?" In Powell and Clemens, *Private Action and the Public Good,* 36–46.

Wood, Allen W. "Exploitation." *Social Philosophy and Policy* 12, no. 2 (1995): 136–58.

Wuthnow, Robert. *Acts of Compassion: Caring for Others and Helping Ourselves.* Princeton: Princeton University Press, 1991.

———. *Learning to Care: Elementary Kindness in an Age of Indifference.* New York: Oxford University Press, 1995.

———. *Poor Richard's Principle: Recovering the American Dream through the Moral Dimension of Work, Business and Money.* Princeton: Princeton University Press, 1996.

Yomtoob, Parichehr, and Ted Schwarz. *The Gift of Life.* New York: St. Martin's Press, 1986.

Younger, Stuart J., Renée Fox, and Laurence J. O'Connell, eds. *Organ Transplantation: Meanings and Realities.* Madison: University of Wisconsin Press, 1996.

Zaner, Richard M., ed. *Death: Beyond Whole-Brain Criteria.* Boston: Kluwer Academic Publishers, 1988.

Zelizer, Viviana. "Beyond the Polemics of the Market: Establishing a Theoretical and Empirical Agenda." *Sociological Forum* 3 (1988): 614–34.

———. "Human Values and the Market: The Case of Life-Insurance and Death in 19th Century America." *American Journal of Sociology* 84 (1978): 591–610.

———. *Morals and Markets: The Development of Life Insurance in the United States.* New York: Columbia University Press, 1979.

———. "The Purchase of Intimacy." *Law and Social Inquiry* 25, no. 3 (2000): 817–48.

———. *The Social Meaning of Money.* New York: Basic Books, 1994.

Zimmerman, D., S. Donnelly, J. Miller, D. Stewart, and S. E. Albert. "Gender Disparity in Living Renal Transplant Donation." *American Journal of Kidney Diseases* 36, no. 3 (2000): 534–40.

Index